'Learning to be a doctor is not just about swinging a steth. shaking a test tube. It is also about learning how to talk to people, and how to understand emotions – those experienced by both the patient and the doctor. Student psychotherapy schemes play an important role in developing these essential skills. They also can be an important rite of passage as the student starts to mature into the doctor. Certainly in my own education I remember that this was the first time in my student career that my teachers were interested in my own opinions, and not just as a way of showing me how wrong they were, and the first time I was given a real, and not fake, task to complete and responsibility to assume. It was one of the reasons that I, and many other students exposed to similar experiences, decided that psychiatry might be for me. I strongly believe that every medical school in the land should host a Student Psychotherapy Scheme, and this book tells you both how and why.' — **Professor Simon Wessely, President of the Royal College of Psychiatrists**

'This lively book is clearly written and illustrated with freshly described, first-hand accounts from students who have been therapists or group participants, and doctors who have been supervisors or Balint leaders in the University College Student Psychotherapy or student Balint group schemes. The authors argue that this approach complements the now routine core communication skills teaching for medical students, and the vignettes certainly make the case that the experience encourages students to think about their own emotional responses as well as the patient's state of mind.' — **Professor Patricia Hughes, Dean for Staff and Student Affairs, Professor of Psychiatry and Education, St. George's, University of London, UK**

'In learning to listen, doctors need to recognise and understand their emotional responses to patients. Medical schools do now include some communication skills training but this cuts little ice in the face of the old institutionalised mantra, "don't get involved". This excellent and timely book describes the schemes developed by University College over many years in which students are introduced to thinking more deeply about the emotional experience of their clinical work. The present volume will be invaluable to all those involved in establishing similar schemes in other medical schools, as well as to students, tutors, general practitioners, psychiatrists and psychotherapists who remain committed to improving this aspect of medical training.' — **Dr Andrew Elder, FRCGP, Consultant in General Practice and Primary Care, UK**

Learning about Emotions in Illness

Good communication between the doctor and patient is essential for the patient to establish a trusting relationship with their doctor and to make the best use of the appropriate treatment. Traditional methods for teaching communication skills have focused on simulated clinical situations in which students learn how to improve their communication, with actors playing the part of the patients, rather than from live experiences with patients. Psychodynamic psychotherapy, with its emphasis on learning to reflect on experiences, offers the student the possibility of learning from a real experience with a patient. Such opportunities allow students to learn directly about patients' emotions, as well as to appreciate their own emotional responses to illness and to communicate better with their patients.

In this book, Peter Shoenberg, Jessica Yakeley and their contributors, who include students and teachers, discuss two different teaching approaches developed at University College London to help medical students understand the role of emotions in illness, communicate more effectively and gain a deeper understanding of the doctor–patient relationship. The benefits of Ball, Wolff and Tredgold's Student Psychotherapy Scheme are considered alongside Shoenberg and Suckling's short-term student Balint discussion group scheme to provide clear guidance about how psychotherapeutic understanding can be used to inform medical education, with positive results.

At a time when medicine is becoming increasingly technological and there is a growing demand by the public for more psychologically minded doctors, this book will be a key resource for physicians, general practitioners, psychologists, psychiatrists and psychotherapists who are involved in medical teaching, and for medical students.

Peter Shoenberg is Honorary Consultant Psychiatrist in Psychotherapy at the Camden Psychodynamic Psychotherapy Service for the Camden and Islington NHS Foundation Trust, UK. He is involved in running student Balint discussion groups and supervising students on the Student Psychotherapy Scheme at University College London, UK.

Jessica Yakeley is Consultant Psychiatrist in Forensic Psychotherapy at the Portman Clinic and Associate Medical Director and Director of Medical Education at the Tavistock and Portman NHS Foundation Trust, UK.

Explorations in Mental Health series

Learning about Emotions in Illness

Integrating psychotherapeutic teaching into medical education

Edited by Peter Shoenberg and Jessica Yakeley

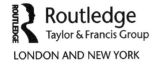

Routledge
Taylor & Francis Group

LONDON AND NEW YORK

First published 2014
by Routledge
27 Church Road, Hove, East Sussex, BN3 2FA, UK

and by Routledge
711 Third Avenue, New York, NY 10017

Routledge is an imprint of the Taylor and Francis Group, an informa business

First issued in paperback 2015

British Library Cataloguing in Publication Data
A catalogue record for this book is available from the British Library

Library of Congress Cataloging in Publication Data
Learning about emotions in illness : integrating psychotherapeutic teaching
in medical education / edited by Peter Shoenberg and Jessica Yakeley.
     pages cm. — (Explorations in mental health)
Includes bibliographical references and index.
1. Psychodynamic psychotherapy—Study and teaching. 2. Psychotherapists—
Training of. 3. Psychotherapist and patient. I. Shoenberg, Peter, editor of
compilation. II. Yakeley, Jessica, 1963- editor of compilation.
RC489.P72.L43 2014
616.89'140076—dc23   2013038037

ISBN 978-0-415-64490-7 (hbk)
ISBN 978-1-138-18911-9 (pbk)
ISBN 978-0-203-07889-1 (ebk)

Typeset in Bembo
by Keystroke, Station Road, Codsall, Wolverhampton

Contents

Contributors

Dr Ray Brown MA FRCPsych is a psychoanalytic psychotherapist and an Honorary Senior Lecturer in Community Medicine at Bristol University and was formerly a Consultant Psychiatrist in Psychotherapy at Callington Road Hospital, and the Psychological Therapies Service, Petherton Resource Centre, Bristol.

Dr Robbie Bunt BSc MRCGP is a General Practitioner Principal at the River Place Health Centre, London.

Dr Lara Curran MB BS BSc is a Foundation Year 1 doctor at University College London Hospital, London.

Dr Elsa Gubert MA MRCGP is a General Practitioner at the Cloister Road Surgery, London.

Dr Caroline Hulsker MA MB BS is a Paediatric Surgery trainee at Great Ormond Street Hospital for Children, London.

Dr Jennifer Johns MB BS DRCOG is a psychoanalyst and former Clinical Assistant in Psychotherapy in the Department of Psychotherapy at University College Hospital, London. She was previously a General Practioner for many years.

Dr Noah Moran MB BS is an Obstetrics and Gynaecology trainee in Merseyside.

Professor Gary Rodin FRCPC MD is Head of Psychosocial Oncology and Palliative Care at the Princess Margaret Hospital, University Health Network, Toronto and was formerly Head of the Department of Psychiatry at the Toronto General Hospital. He is also a psychoanalyst.

Dr Paul Sackin FRCGP is a retired General Practitioner and former President of the Balint Society. He is an Honorary Specialist Doctor at the Camden Psychodynamic Psychotherapy Service (formerly the UCLH and Royal Free Hospital Departments of Psychotherapy), London.

Dr Peter Shoenberg MA MRCP (UK) FRCPsych is Honorary Consultant Psychiatrist in Psychotherapy at the Camden Psychodynamic Psychotherapy Service (formerly the UCLH and Royal Free Hospital Departments of Psychotherapy) for the Camden and Islington NHSFoundation Trust, UK, London. He was formerly Head of the Department of Psychotherapy at University College London Hospital and Honorary Senior Clinical Lecturer in Psychiatry at University College London Medical School. He is also a psychoanalytic psychotherapist.

Dr Heather Suckling FRCGP is a retired GP and former President of the Balint Society and Secretary of the International Balint Federation. She is a part time Tutor in Professional Development at University College London Medical School and an Honorary Specialist Doctor at the Camden Psychodynamic Pyschotherapy Service (formerly the UCLH and Royal Free Hospital Departments of Psychotherapy), London.

Dr Thanos Tsapas MRCPsych MSc is Consultant Psychiatrist in Psychotherapy at Callington Road Hospital, Bristol and the Psychological Therapies Service, Petherton Resource Centre, Bristol.

Dr Christine Van Duuren MB BS is a Specialist Doctor in Psychiatry in Psychotherapy at the Camden Psychodynamic Psychotherapy Service (formerly the UCLH and Royal Free Hospital Departments of Psychotherapy), London. She is also a psychoanalytic psychotherapist.

Dr Jessica Yakeley MA MRCP(UK) FRCPsych is Consultant Psychiatrist in Forensic Psychotherapy at the Portman Clinic and Associate Medical Director and Director of Medical Education at the Tavistock and Portman NHS Foundation Trust, UK. She was Consultant Psychiatrist in Psychotherapy at the Camden Psychodynamic Psychotherapy Service from 2003 to 2010. She is also a psychoanalyst.

Dr Sotiris Zalidis MRCP(UK) is a General Practitioner Principal at the Well Street Surgery in London and formerly a Member of the Council of the Balint Society. He is an Honorary Specialist Doctor at the Camden Psychodynamic Psychotherapy Service (formerly the UCLH and Royal Free Hospital Departments of Psychotherapy), London.

Foreword

This text, *Learning about Emotions in Illness*, edited by Peter Shoenberg and Jessica Yakeley, is an important and unique contribution to the literature on medical education. It is also pleasing to me, in both personal and professional ways, to see its publication. I was fortunate to have met Peter Shoenberg more than two decades ago when he visited Canada and to have been introduced at that time to the UCL Student Psychotherapy Scheme. I have been fascinated to observe its evolution over time and to witness first-hand the sensitive and skilful process of supervision when I later sat in on Shoenberg's group supervision of students at University College London. I was equally impressed when David Sturgeon later brought with him to the Toronto General Hospital a most remarkable group of students who were participating in the scheme at the time. Unable to hide behind theory, which they had not yet learned, and too junior to have become cynical and disillusioned, these students brought their humanity to the clinical interaction in a way that deeply impressed us all. My first thought was that somehow the scheme had attracted the most exceptional British medical students, but now realise that this program had allowed the compassion and empathic understanding of these talented students to emerge in a creative and constructive way. They became able to see the whole person they were treating, not just the disease or the symptom complex. They were privileged to have received the most important learning experience of all in medicine at this very early stage of their career.

The Student Psychotherapy Scheme is a response to a problem that needed to be fixed. Indeed, there has been a growing awareness in medical education that neither undergraduate nor postgraduate training has adequately prepared physicians for the complex and demanding task of attending to the emotional needs of their patients (Buckman et al., 2011). Those who enter the speciality of psychiatry may receive more training at that time, but the large majority of medical graduates who enter general practice or other medical specialties have been inadequately prepared for this task. Traditional medical education has emphasised the technical and factual aspects of medical care, presumably based on the assumption that the necessary skills in establishing therapeutic and effective physician–patient relationships would automatically be acquired or else learned through a mysterious osmotic process. Evidence suggests that this is not the case. In fact, a recent systematic review of research in that area indicates that empathy typically declines over the course of both undergraduate and postgraduate education (Neumann et al., 2011). Other research suggests that 'empathic opportunities' in clinical interviews are most often overlooked by practitioners (Pollak et al., 2007). This deficiency in medical practice may be due to multiple factors, including clinical volumes, the structure of health care delivery and the lack of adequate training. When support is not provided to students to help them process their experience with patients in highly distressing circumstances, emotional overload, exhaustion and avoidance of emotions in clinical interactions may result.

The Student Psychotherapy Scheme was initiated as a small project at University College London more than 50 years ago by Dorothea Ball, Heinz Wolff and Roger Tredgold. Many other students and faculty have been involved in the project since that time, some of whom are contributors to this text. Yakeley herself was a student in the scheme, supervised by Shoenberg, with whom she co-edited the text. Students and faculty who were involved with the scheme at different stages in its evolution over the years have contributed to the rich tapestry that is provided in the description of the scheme in this text from multiple and different perspectives. The influence of the scheme is also evident in the emergence of similar programmes at other centres in England, Europe and Canada, and in the testimony of so many medical practitioners of its lasting impact upon their career and clinical practice.

In its approach, the scheme avoids the common problem of students in formal psychotherapy and psychoanalytic training programmes, which is that the teaching of theory interferes with the process of empathic engagement. Although theoretical training is important for psychotherapy practitioners, its early introduction may actually diminish the extent to which junior trainees are able to situate themselves within the emotional lives of their patients. The Student Psychotherapy Scheme begins with an early emphasis on empathic engagement and receptive listening. This approach helps to allow a powerful human experience to emerge between patient and student therapist, upon which later theoretical understanding can be built.

It is humbling for experienced therapists, who place value on the intensive, often lengthy, training in theory and in practice that they have undertaken to observe that excellent results can be obtained with supervised student therapists who have no prior formal training in psychotherapy. It is particularly striking to observe this in the Student Psychotherapy Scheme, where the supervision takes place in a group setting rather than on an individual basis, where there can be a more detailed discussion of the process of most or all sessions. The success for supervised student therapists, however, should not be taken to indicate that advanced training in psychotherapy is unimportant. Rather, it may demonstrate that good outcomes can occur with student therapists when cases are well selected, when there is an experienced supervisor and when the goals of treatment are limited and short term. Evidence from the psychotherapy outcome research literature suggests that although the experience of a therapist predicts positive outcomes (Scott et al., 2005), active engagement of the therapist is a significant predictor of short-term positive outcomes (Heinonen et al., 2012).

The intent of the Student Psychotherapy Scheme is to enhance its trainees awareness and sensitivity to the emotional lives of their patients and themselves, with particular attention to the doctor–patient relationship. This is achieved by examining, in a supervised group format, the experience of the students who have taken on patients in a psychotherapeutic treatment. This is a powerful and valuable experience for the participating students, but the requirement to find suitable cases can be a limiting factor in the growth and extension of such programmes. Further, the learning from psychotherapy cases must be extrapolated to the range of clinical interactions in which undergraduate medical students find themselves.

The UCL group extended their training programme by establishing so-called Balint groups. This approach, promulgated by Hungarian-born British psychoanalyst Michael Balint, involves supervised group meetings of doctors to discuss the psychodynamic aspects of their relationships with patients. Such groups are conducted to allow physicians to share their experience and to apply psychodynamic principles across the range of clinical practice. The personal vignettes reported by the students and Balint leaders in this text capture the range of perplexing personal, clinical and ethical dilemmas that physicians and students may struggle with in the course of clinical care.

Although high work-load is often cited as an important factor contributing to physician burnout (Brown & Gunderman, 2006), it is equally possible that it is the failure of empathy (Zenasni et al., 2012) and of managing the difficult emotions that are evoked in clinical situations (Shanafelt & Dyrbye, 2012) that contributes to burnout. Balint groups provide an opportunity for students to understand and manage these emotions by reflecting on their experience in diverse clinical situations. This unique contribution of Balint groups to medical education may account for their growing incorporation into medical undergraduate teaching programs in many parts of the world. The feasibility of such groups allows this experience to be available to students who could not otherwise access the Student Psychotherapy Scheme.

There are now many courses on communication that have been initiated for medical undergraduates, postgraduates and medical practitioners and evidence suggests that such training improves the skills of students and physicians in empathic communication (Buckman et al., 2011). However, the use of the term 'communication', which literally refers to the exchange of information, may still reflect the emphasis in medicine on action, rather than on emotional receptivity. Notably, this text is squarely focused on learning about emotions in illness, through participating in two schemes which provide a longitudinal experience. Although there may now be seminars on communication in many medical schools and postgraduate training programmes, experts in medical education tell us that learning is most effective when it is contextual, ongoing and affectively engaging.

Throughout the text and, particularly in Yakeley's summary of research in Chapter 8, evidence is presented to demonstrate that the Student Psychotherapy Scheme has been helpful to the patients and to the students in the development of their psychotherapeutic skills, their emotional maturity and their subsequent career paths, and that the new student Balint scheme also enhances students' emotional maturity. Clearly both schemes give them a deeper understanding of the doctor–patient relationship. Although there may be an association between participating in the Student Psychotherapy Scheme and a subsequent decision to pursue training in psychiatry, an even more powerful indicator of the impact of this scheme is the extent to which those who have participated in the scheme have communicated how powerfully it has affected their personal and professional development.

In some respects, the Student Psychotherapy Scheme and the student Balint group scheme have emerged in response to the increasing specialisation of medicine, and its growing dependence on technology, with fewer opportunities for trainees to develop and maintain longitudinal relationships with patients. In a similar way, the field of palliative care developed in reaction to the failure of mainstream medicine to address the emotional and physical suffering of patients with advanced disease and their families (Clark, 2007). Although expensive technology was available in many well-resourced settings, there was a relative neglect of training and care to support the emotional well-being of patients and the control of their symptoms. The recent rise of interest in the support of the spiritual well-being of medical patients reflects this perceived need to draw attention to the whole person, including their subjective well-being, in the delivery of medical care (Lo et al., 2011). Spiritual well-being has been defined in this context as the extent to which individuals are at peace with themselves, feel their lives have meaning and purpose, and derive comfort from their beliefs in the face of suffering (Canada et al., 2008). Although religion and other belief systems may contribute to this outcome, it can also be enhanced by the creation of reflective space in a relationship of a patient with a health care provider. The Student Psychotherapy Scheme helps students to create such reflective space for patients who might otherwise experience feelings of overwhelming distress and isolation.

It is a rare pleasure to observe the growth over several decades of an idea and then a programme that has the potential to make fundamental change in the practice of medicine. Peter Shoenberg has been an important leader and steward of the two schemes, helping to ensure their innovation, continuity and dissemination. The text is a testament to their lasting value and impact on the professional and personal lives of so many people. The contributors have communicated convincingly that emotions are central to human psychological life and well-being, and that learning about emotions in illness must be a central component of any medical curriculum. More importantly, they have developed an approach to such education that is meaningful, practical and transportable to diverse medical settings.

Gary Rodin

Acknowledgements

We would like to thank our predecessors, Dorothea Ball, Heinz Wolff and Roger Tredgold who started the Student Psychotherapy Scheme and Michael Balint who started the first student Balint group at University College Hospital. Those of us who were taught by them were deeply inspired to carry on the tradition that they established over 50 years ago. That this first scheme has continued until the present day and that the later student Balint groups have thrived owes much to the enthusiastic participation over many years of generations of medical students 'who taught us how to teach' (Wolff et al., 1990) and to the Student Psychotherapy Scheme administrative secretary Valerie Fenn, who got to know each of the student psychotherapists individually and helped them to feel safe in their work with patients in our Department of Psychotherapy. We also thank all the members of staff who participated in our schemes either as psychotherapy supervisors or as Balint leaders, especially David Sturgeon who was so vital for the early and subsequent development of the UCL Student Psychotherapy Scheme. We also thank Abe Brafman, Fakhry Davids and Ronnie Doctor, who led discussion groups for students on their psychiatric attachments, which helped us to develop the idea of short-term student Balint groups at UCL, and the Melanie Klein and Winnicott Trusts, which supported this earlier project. We are very grateful to the medical school at University College London, in particular Margaret Lloyd and Deborah Gill, who consistently supported our two schemes and helped us to develop and finance the student Balint groups in recent years, and Camden and Islington NHS Foundation Trust, which created a new Consultant Medical Psychotherapist post to run and research these schemes. The UK Balint Society, which has been an invaluable support for our student Balint group project, has also given us a regular forum to discuss our work.

Many people have helped in the preparation of this book and we would especially like to thank Jonathan Silverman, who gave wise advice about communication skills teaching, and Erika Drucker, George Freeman, Sue Gagg, Jane Gatrell, Marnie Hodgkin, Dick Joyce, David and Christie Lane, Heide Otten, Zhenia Shoenberg and John Turner who read and made helpful comments on parts of our manuscript. Ray Brown and Thanos Tsapas, the authors of Chapter 4 about the Bristol Student Psychotherapy Scheme, would also like to thank David Mumford whose involvement and educational perspective was vital in establishing this scheme in Bristol. In addition they would like to thank all the students who participated in their scheme over the past 16 years for their enthusiasm, commitment and creativity and to also thank Gloria Babiker, Paul Curtis, Simon Downer, Kristina Gintalaite, Ami Kothari, Alice Lomax, David Porteous, Geoff Van der Linden, Thuli Whitehouse, Polly Wood and Maureen Wright.

We are grateful to Johanna Shapiro for allowing us to draw on her article published in *Academic Medicine* (2011) in the Introduction and to the UK Balint Society for permission to quote extensively from articles by Shoenberg (2012), Moran (2009) and Curran (2011) published in the *Journal of the Balint Society* in Chapters 5 and 7 and to the *Bulletin of the Romanian Balint Society* to quote in Chapter 5 from the paper by Suckling (2005). The quotation in the Conclusion from an excerpt of a student's psychotherapy summary was originally printed in the *Journal of the Balint Society* and subsequently in *Psychosomatics: The Uses of Psychotherapy* (Shoenberg, 2007) and is reproduced with the permission of Libby Salnow, the UK Balint Society and Palgrave Macmillan. The full published version of this is available from Palgrave Macmillan. Last but not least we are indebted to all the patients who either took part in the UCL and Bristol Student Psychotherapy Schemes or who were reflected on in the student Balint group discussions, whose stories (which are anonymised so that that they are not identifiable) are told in this book. Without them none of this would have been possible.

Introduction

Peter Shoenberg

> I've never talked to a patient before. It could be someone's grandmother
> or wife . . . I should be able to take a history from them – I've got a book
> which tells me what questions to ask – but I don't know how to do it . . .
> I've never failed a test before and I feel I may fail this one . . . Everyone just
> says, 'You'll get used to it'.
>
> Roger, a medical student quoted in *Making Doctors.*
> *An Institutional Apprenticeship*, p. 199 by Simon Sinclair (1997)

Medical students beginning their clinical studies go through a psychological
transition from being passive recipients of academic knowledge to becoming
active participants in the clinical world of the hospital. They are no longer free
agents in a safe academic environment, but are now faced with illness and
patients, and find themselves at the bottom of the hierarchy in a teaching hospital, where they must learn to acquire a new professional role. How will they
cope with this major change and what sort of relationship will they develop
with the patients they see? How are they to deal with the many emotions they
witness in their patients, as well as with their own emotional reactions to these
patients and with being confronted by distressing clinical situations?

Shapiro (2011) describes various studies concerning students' emotional
responses to patients, pointing out that emotional distress in students is
common (Rhodes-Kropf et al., 2005): students, when faced with serious illness
and death, report feelings of helplessness and uncertainty; they find their initial
attempts at physical examination anxiety provoking and are afraid of being
humiliated by hospital staff (Pitkala and Mantyranta, 2003; 2004). First-year
clinical medical students are distressed by anxiety, guilt, sadness, anger and
shame triggered by their uncertainty, powerlessness and conflicts of values
(Beca et al., 2007). Sadly, they often view their own emotions with suspicion:
students consider crying in front of patients or colleagues to be unprofessional
(Sung et al., 2009). Although students want to establish emotional connections
with patients (Rucker and Shapiro, 2003), they are frightened of being overwhelmed by their feelings towards patients (Shapiro, 2011; Bombeke et al.,
2010). When they witness physicians dealing with their own anxiety by

distancing themselves from their own feelings (Ahluwalia et al., 2010), students may try to emulate their teachers and begin to deal with their own difficult emotions in the same way.

One study, which measured empathy in US medical students throughout their training, found a significant and worrying decline in empathy scores during the first clinical year which persisted until graduation (Hojat et al., 2009). However, this study used a measure of empathy relying on a cognitive definition of empathy and such a decline was not observed in similar studies using the same measure made in Japan (Kataoka et al., 2009) or Korea (Roh et al., 2010). In spite of medical schools' attempts to encourage human qualities in their students, cynicism often seems to develop (Kay, 1990; Silver and Glicken, 1990; Sheehan et al., 1990; Wolf et al., 1989).

We know that good communication between a doctor and patient allows a trusting relationship to develop, so that the patient can make the best use of the medical encounter. It helps the patient to feel safe enough to speak about the psychological aspects of their story, so that there can be a shared understanding of the patient's emotional as well as physical problems. As medicine becomes more specialised and dependent on technology, the need for this kind of communication is more pressing. Communication inevitably includes dealing with an emotional component. Medical students must learn about communication skills and about the role of emotions in illness to become effective as future doctors. Our book is about two psychotherapy teaching methods which can help medical students learn about the role of emotions in illness. The first method offers students the opportunity for each to see a patient for one year of weekly psychodynamic psychotherapy. The second method, drawing on the work of the psychoanalyst Michael Balint, offers students the opportunity to speak in a weekly discussion group about their initial experiences of being with patients.

When students start clinical studies, for the first time they regularly encounter severe illness, disfigurement, emotional distress and death and dying. They may have strong emotional reactions to such experiences, which may be difficult to manage and lead to defensive strategies to deal with the impact of what they see. They observe the behaviour of their teachers and other clinical staff. Much good teaching about communication skills can still be provided at the bedside, where students are influenced by doctors who show sensitive and caring approaches to their patients. Unfortunately there is often 'a hidden curriculum' in medical education (Hafferty, 1998), in which students are exposed to less satisfactory role modelling: as they progress through medical school, their prior sensitive attitudes may be replaced by cooler more detached ones towards patients, especially if they identify with the less emotional approaches of some of their seniors. Of course students have to acquire some emotional detachment needed for effective clinical decision making and actions, but they also need to stay enough in touch with their emotions to be empathic towards their patients.

Certain clinical attachments, such as general practice and psychiatry, traditionally give students special opportunities to learn about communication skills (Whitehouse, 2009). In both disciplines much emphasis is put on understanding the social and psychological background of the patient. In general practice, which espouses a psychosomatic approach, students have the possibility of considering emotional factors in medical illness and of learning to reflect on the consultations they observe. In psychiatry, students learn how to conduct in-depth psychological interviews, as well as recognise depression and deal with common psychiatric emergencies, such as suicidal or acutely psychotic patients.

In the apprenticeship model of medical teaching, students during their clinical studies are attached to one or two clinical teachers for some weeks at a time and learn clinical medicine by following up patients on the ward. This gives the students an opportunity to build a relationship with their patients, while studying their diseases; but as hospital inpatient stays get shorter and there are increasing numbers of students at each medical school, these possibilities for individual student–patient relationships have diminished.

Medical students often struggle to find their place within the vast hierarchy of the teaching hospital and to learn how to develop a new professional role (including its boundaries) in these encounters with patients. They are under pressure to absorb enormous amounts of new information and to learn the rules of routine clinical procedures (e.g. performing a careful physical examination). Many are at a stage in their own personal development where they are independent for the first time in their life and beginning to explore new relationships of their own as adults. To learn about the emotional experiences of patients and the students' emotional responses to them, students need a safe and non-judgemental setting in which their patients' and their own feelings can be reflected on and in which they can speak freely about the relationship between themselves and their patients. Psychodynamic psychotherapeutic teaching may offer some solutions to this problem.

We know that many physical illnesses can be precipitated by emotional events and some (e.g. the somatoform disorders) are caused by an underlying emotional disturbance in the patient (Shoenberg, 2007). Patients' emotions may significantly influence their clinical outcomes (van Middendorp et al., 2010; Kurlander et al., 2009; Gazmararian et al., 2009) and the doctor–patient relationship. Yet, as Shapiro has pointed out (2011), medical students often feel embarrassed and uncomfortable when confronted with these emotions (Benbasset and Baumal, 2001) and may see patients' negative emotions as a barrier to a patient-centred approach (Bower et al., 2009).

Full appreciation of the range of emotions experienced by patients with different illnesses requires a teaching approach that involves the student in reflecting on live encounters with patients. Recognition of their own emotional responses to being with ill patients can be best learned from such live experiences: the feelings of guilt and anger aroused by an angry patient, or the sadness and helplessness felt in dealing with a terminally ill patient, cannot be easily reproduced in a simulated situation. Students are more likely to develop appropriate empathy by understanding their own emotional responses to real illnesses and patients. Hence the title of this book: *Learning about Emotions in Illness*.

Communication skills teaching

In British medical education there has always been a strong emphasis on the importance of clinical skills, reflected in the priority they are given in the final professional exams. Yet until relatively recently, the aspects of clinical skills concerned with communication were often poorly defined within the curriculum and not directly assessed. In 1985, the Nuffield Provincial Hospitals Trust publication *Talking with patients: A teaching approach* advocated the idea of teaching communication skills in medical schools.

In the 1980s important evidence about the need for such teaching was building up. It was found that psychosocial and psychiatric problems were being missed in up to 50% of cases in general medical practice (Schulberg and Burns, 1988; Freeling et al., 1985) and that most complaints by the general public about doctors were to do with communication problems rather than clinical competency issues (Shapiro et al., 1989). Patient anxiety and dissatisfaction were related to uncertainty and lack of information, explanation and feedback from the doctor (Faden et al., 1981; Mackillop et al., 1988; Frances et al., 1969). In one study patients were interrupted by their doctor so soon after they began describing their presenting problem that they failed to disclose other significant concerns (Beckman and Frankel, 1984). The quality of clinical communication was found to be related to positive health outcomes: studies showed that reduction of blood pressure was significantly greater in patients whose doctors allowed them to express health concerns without interruption (Orth et al., 1987). Explaining and understanding patient concerns, even when they could not be resolved, resulted in a significant fall in anxiety (MacLeod, 1991). Cultural differences also were found to interfere with communication (Simpson, 1980). Eventually, *The Toronto Consensus Statement* (Simpson et al., 1991) argued that, since problems in doctor–patient communication were so common and had such a demonstrably adverse effect on patient management, there was sufficient evidence to support the incorporation of the teaching of communication skills into medical school curricula.

Since then there has been a revolution in teaching communication skills in the UK (Whitehouse, 2009), so that now all 33 medical schools have included this in their curriculum. The General Medical Council (2002), the British Medical Association (2003) and the Department of Health (2003, 2004) all advocated that the teaching and assessment of clinical communication skills should become a central component of undergraduate medical education in the UK. The UK Consensus statement on the content of communication curricula in undergraduate medical education (von Fragstein et al., 2008) recognised six domains of communication learning, which were:

1   Respect for others.
2   Awareness of the evidence base for good communication skills.
3   Learning the tasks of clinical communication.
4   Handling specific issues (e.g. handling emotions, dealing with uncertainty, dealing with communication impairment, age-specific issues, cultural and social diversity, handling mistakes and complaints, sensitive issues and specific application of explanation).
5   Learning to communicate using different media (e.g. telephone, computer).
6   Learning to communicate beyond the patient (e.g. with relatives or carers, or with interpreters).

The most popular communication skills teaching approach in the UK is the Calgary-Cambridge Guide to the medical interview, developed by Kurtz, Silverman, and Draper (2005) (Silverman et al., 2005; Silverman, 2009) and now used in about 70% of British medical schools. It defines the following aims for the doctor–patient consultation: (1) Initiating the session, (2) Gathering information, (3) Providing structure to the consultation, (4) Building the relationship, (5) Explanation and planning, and (6) Closing the session. The amount and timing of teaching[1] may vary: in some medical schools the main skills are taught in the first 2 years of study, but in many they are taught during the last 3 years, when students have most contact with their patients.

Such communication skills are now taught in medical schools in many countries in Europe and in North America and Australia. Although these teaching methods have radically changed the way many students think about patients, they are often based on experiences with simulated patients. Communication skills teaching may not show students how to recognise patients' feelings, even if it helps them to become more aware of those situations where difficulties in communication are likely to arise, and to learn strategies to deal with these. For the student to fully understand and appreciate their patients' emotions, these have to be experienced in a live situation (Hojat, 2009). Psychodynamic psychotherapy teaching offers medical students important opportunities for achieving this goal.[2]

Psychodynamic psychotherapy teaching

As Michael Balint, who developed discussion groups for GPs (Balint groups), observed, the psychotherapist is in a unique position to help medical students develop new insights into their relationships with patients and reflect on the links between emotions and physical symptoms. Psychodynamic psycho-therapeutic teaching, with its emphasis on learning to reflect on experience, can help the student to learn about patients' emotions and to better appreciate their own emotional responses to illness.

Traditionally, this is given as part of the psychiatric teaching in the form of lectures or tutorials, in which students learn about the uses of this type of therapy and its theoretical basis. Students are taught about the role of the unconscious in normal and abnormal behaviour, the role of defence mechanisms in human relationships (Crisp, 1986) and about the importance of a secure early attachment. In some departments students may observe psychodynamic therapy through a one-way mirror. Role play also may be used. In our department at UCL students sit in on psychotherapy assessments of patients from whom they have taken a history.

The UCL Student Psychotherapy Scheme

Fifty years ago Dorothea Ball and Heinz Wolff, psychiatrists at University College Hospital, allowed some of the first-year clinical medical students at UCL to follow up a patient in once weekly individual psychodynamic psychotherapy over 1 year, with the aim of helping to learn about the doctor–patient relationship (Ball and Wolff, 1963; Shoenberg, 1992). In the UCL Student Psychotherapy Scheme that has evolved since that time, each student sees his or her patient alone and is given weekly supervision in a group of fellow students by a senior member of staff. The treatment is offered to the patient as an introduction to psychodynamic psychotherapy. The students find this a deeply engaging experience and to patients the students' gentle and sensitive approach is very helpful, especially for those with milder personality and psychosomatic disorders.

We have found that this scheme helps medical students to learn how to listen to their patients, to tolerate and handle the difficult emotions arising in the patient and themselves, and to understand the significance of their patient's early emotional life and its relationship to their current symptoms. Above all, students experience a professional relationship with a patient, in which the patient's dependency needs can be understood and valued and they learn about the importance of continuity of care during a time when most of their contact with patients is fragmentary. Such long-term psychotherapy experiences are deeply rewarding for the students and patients alike. Students are learning from these live encounters about their patients' emotions and how to reflect on their emotional responses to patients. In the chapters that follow, written by supervisors and students who participated in the scheme, many examples of such clinical experiences are given that show just how rewarding this experience can be.

Medical student Balint discussion groups

Because of the limited number of suitable patients and available supervisors, we were never able to take more than a handful of new students (10 to 15) each year into our psychotherapy scheme. When our medical school doubled its intake of medical students in 2003, we wanted to find new ways of helping students to learn about the doctor–patient relationship. We therefore introduced a modified form of student Balint discussion group for first-year clinical medical students to talk about their experiences with patients (Shoenberg and Suckling, 2004). Balint himself had developed such student discussion groups at UCL in the late 1960s with two longer-term weekly groups (Balint et al., 1969).

We offered students a discussion group which met for 1 hour each week over 12 weeks. Each group was led by a GP who was a qualified Balint leader, together with a medically qualified senior psychotherapist. At the beginning of each group, one of the leaders asked if any student had a patient who had remained in their mind, whom they would like to discuss. After the presentation the other students were encouraged to comment on the story. In this way we looked at the feelings aroused in the student by the patient and explored the relationship of the student with the patient. This proved to be a most rewarding experience and our modified shorter-term groups proved very popular with the students and eventually became an option on the curriculum. Now up to 100 students each year can participate in these groups, which help them learn about their own and their patients' emotions and about the doctor–patient relationship.

An outline of the book

In Chapter 1, Jessica Yakeley describes the development of the UCL Student Psychotherapy Scheme and its impact on students' learning about the doctor–patient relationship. In Chapter 2, Christine Van Duuren and Jennifer Johns write about their experience of supervising medical students on this scheme. In Chapter 3, four doctors (Jessica Yakeley, Robbie Bunt, Elsa Gubert and Caroline Hulsker) who originally participated in this scheme, write about their experiences of seeing patients on our UCL Student Psychotherapy Scheme and how these have influenced them in their subsequent careers. In Chapter 4, Ray Brown and Thanos Tsapas describe some of the problems of setting up a similar scheme at the University of Bristol.

In Chapter 5, Heather Suckling and I describe the UCL student Balint discussion group scheme and assess its impact on the students' thinking about their emotional responses to their patients. In Chapter 6, Sotiris Zalidis, one of our student Balint group leaders, writes about the students' problems of professional identity and boundary confusion and how the Balint group can help them with these difficulties. In Chapter 7 two former Balint group students (Noah Moran and Lara Curran) write about their experiences of participating in a group and a GP (Paul Sackin) reflects on his experience in Michael Balint's original student group. In Chapter 8, Jessica Yakeley writes about our research on the impact of these two teaching methods on students and their patients. The Conclusion is written by me.

As teachers and students, we continue to find these psychotherapeutic experiences inspiring and encouraging. We believe that communication skills teaching, while a vital part of the medical curriculum, can be much enhanced by the teaching methods we describe (Crisp, 1986). These teaching methods help students develop their own empathic responses to their patients by helping them to think about their own and their patients' emotions in illness.

Notes

1   For example, at Cambridge University, communication skills teaching is integrated into the clinical course so that students receive a half day of communication skills teaching on a difficult situation, relevant to the speciality they are studying on their current clinical attachment. Included in the final exams is a simulated clinical encounter exam, which must be passed for the students to qualify as doctors.

2   There are other ways of achieving this goal, such as classroom discussions about emotionally challenging clinical situations, counselling of individual students, and training students to assess their own performance, which can also help students to develop emotional self-awareness (Benbassat and Baumal, 2005). In addition, reflective writing about personal illness narratives (DasGupta and Charon, 2004) can be used to enhance empathy in medical students. This may also be achieved by other methods such as analysing audio- or video-taped encounters, role-play, shadowing a patient, experiencing hospitalisation, or studying literature and the arts (Hojat, 2009). At one medical school students are offered an elective course on the Art of Doctoring (Shapiro, 2011).

Chapter 1

The UCL Student Psychotherapy Scheme[1]

Jessica Yakeley

Introduction

Although motivations for choosing a career in medicine are varied and complex, most medical students start their clinical studies with a commitment to help and care for their patients, often accompanied by a genuine curiosity and openness towards illness and suffering. These attitudes, however, may become quickly challenged by their immersion in a medical culture which implicitly or explicitly discourages emotional attachments to patients and provides limited opportunities to get to know individual patients in any depth. Medical students often complain that their contacts with patients are brief and fragmented with few possibilities of following them through the course of their illness. This makes it difficult for students to gain understanding of how a patient's presenting illness relates to his or her personal history, particularly in its psychological and emotional aspects. Although initiatives at some medical schools, such as following a cancer patient for several months through their treatment (at University College London [UCL] this is called the Cancer Patient Pathways project), have gone some way towards addressing this, students nevertheless may be unprepared for the powerful emotional responses evoked in them by their contact with ill and sometimes dying patients, or patients who may be anxious, silent, hostile or uncooperative. Formal teaching forums within the curriculum in which these universal, but often ignored, affective responses in students can be acknowledged and talked about are lacking.

The UCL Student Psychotherapy Scheme (SPS), currently operating under the aegis of University College London School of Medicine from the Camden Psychodynamic Psychotherapy Service, Camden and Islington Foundation Trust, is a unique method of educating first-year clinical medical students about the doctor–patient relationship in which the teaching focuses on just such emotional and psychological issues. By seeing a carefully selected patient for weekly psychotherapy sessions for at least a year under the supervision of an experienced psychodynamic or psychoanalytic psychotherapist, the student has the experience not only of a long-term intensive contact with a patient, but of exposure to a range of emotional responses and non-verbal communications from the patient. Moreover, he or she will have a regular space, provided by the psychotherapy supervision, in which to learn how to reflect on and manage such emotions – his or her own and the patient's – in the best interests of both. Although student therapists will inevitably learn something about the theory and practice of psychodynamic psychotherapy, the main aim of the scheme is to introduce students to a psychodynamic way of thinking about the doctor–patient relationship and to a form of communication skills which will be useful for their future career as doctors, as well as introducing patients to this type of therapy.

I was a student at the then University College and Middlesex School of Medicine and participated in the SPS in the late 1980s supervised by Peter Shoenberg, who was running the scheme at this time. This experience had a lasting and formative influence on both my choice and course of career as a psychiatrist, and laid the foundations for my later training as a medical psychotherapist and psychoanalyst. Fifteen years later, my first consultant psychiatrist post in psychotherapy was back at University College Hospital running the scheme, as well as actively assessing patients, selecting and supervising the medical students, and researching the impact of the scheme (see Chapter 8). My own involvement in the scheme as organiser, educator, supervisor, researcher, and most fundamentally as participating medical student, continues to be a significant source of professional and personal inspiration and fulfilment. However, the real strength of the scheme, which ensures its continued success, lies in the dedication and commitment of both its participating medical students and its supervisors, who provide a valuable therapeutic experience for patients and a unique teaching opportunity, respectively.

History of the Student Psychotherapy Scheme

The Student Psychotherapy Scheme was founded in 1958 by Heinz Wolff and Dorothea Ball, medically qualified psychotherapists, and Roger Tredgold, a psychiatrist, in the Department of Psychological Medicine at University College Hospital (Ball and Wolff, 1963). Yet even before this, first-year clinical medical students attached to the department were encouraged to play an active part in its work and were the first to see newly referred psychiatric outpatients (Sturgeon, 1983). The student would spend an hour with the patient taking a history, and then present this to the consultant psychiatrist and the other medical students. Following this, the patient would be interviewed by the psychiatrist in the presence of the students, who could ask further questions to clarify the diagnosis and formulate management and treatment. On occasion, the psychiatrist would recommend that the patient have some further interviews to give them the opportunity to talk through some of their difficulties in more detail and it was not unusual for the medical student who had originally clerked the patient to volunteer to do this, and report back individually to the psychiatrist.

Two important issues gradually emerged from this informal arrangement which led to the inception of the scheme. The students found that as the patient spoke more about their difficulties, more covert problems emerged which suggested a possible need for psychotherapy, but this might mean waiting several months before a vacancy arose. The medical students who had been seeing patients and developing a relationship with them began to voice their concerns that this relationship had to be abruptly terminated, leaving the patient waiting for treatment. Some also complained that despite being taught a good deal about psychotherapy they were not allowed to see it in action, as sitting in on therapy sessions was contraindicated for the patient (Ball and Wolff, 1963). This led to a few enterprising and enthusiastic students being allowed to continue to see their patients weekly, so long as every session was reported back to the psychiatrist.

We can see here how these students had discovered two fundamental aspects of the doctor–patient relationship that were to become fundamental principles of the Student Psychotherapy Scheme in learning that:

1   The patient's presenting complaint or conscious understanding of their symptoms and difficulties might conceal less conscious factors which nevertheless play a critical part in the genesis and course of their illness.
2   The importance of continuity of care, which was linked to the concept of attachment. These students discovered that the patient did not want to see different doctors, but wanted to continue to see the person – in this case the medical student – with whom they had developed a trusting relationship; the students themselves also felt frustrated by having to hand the patient over to another person, without being involved in the subsequent course of their treatment and its outcome. Now students could see for themselves that their growing relationship with their patients facilitated the emergence of new information about the patients, throwing light on both the origins of the patients' illnesses, as well as informing their treatment and prognosis.

Tredgold, Ball and Wolff were surprised at how sensitive the students were to the psychodynamic issues of the patient, and how quickly some of them picked up and used psychodynamic principles such as transference and countertransference in their interactions with patients. Although the number of students seeing patients in this way was initially small, knowledge of this unusual initiative gradually spread by word of mouth among the students and their peers, so that increasing numbers came forward to ask if they too could take on a patient for psychotherapy. This soon, however, raised a problem for the psychotherapists of finding enough time for the students to be supervised, and led to the suggestion that they should be supervised in groups.

Ball and Wolff (1963) describe the debate which this provoked. On the one hand, it was argued that individual supervision allowed for a confidential relationship to develop between the student and the supervisor, mirroring the one between the student and patient, where the student's personal anxieties and conflicts could be discussed to some extent. On the other hand, not only was individual supervision more time-intensive, but supervision in a group of three or four students allowed students to share their initial anxieties about seeing a patient, as well as enabling students to experience differences between patients and therapeutic approaches through hearing how their fellow students each handled their own patients.

However, Sturgeon (1983) highlights the deeper anxieties and conflicts between the members of staff in the Department of Psychological Medicine exposed by the push towards group supervision. If group supervision were sanctioned and organised, it would require official acknowledgement and approval of the whole enterprise. Not all members of the department believed that students were capable of safely conducting psychotherapy in the best interest of the patient and therefore did not want to be associated with this practice. Serious concerns were expressed about the possibility of the patient breaking down, or even committing suicide whilst being treated by a student therapist, and parallel concerns were voiced about students whose own disturbance might be revealed by their participation in the scheme. Tredgold, as head of the department, decided to allow group supervision to go ahead, and for the scheme to become a formal teaching option for medical students at UCH, considering it to benefit patients and students. He thought that if a student were to break down it was better that this happened early on in his or her career under conditions of close supervision and support rather than years later when conditions might be less favourable and responsibilities greater. However, the concerns voiced by others in the department were not ignored and have influenced the way in which the scheme has developed over the years.

Group supervision allowed more students to see patients in the department at any one time. Another important change which consolidated the scheme as a formal entity was that some students began to ask whether they could see a patient who might be suitable for psychotherapy, but one whom they had not initially clerked (Sturgeon, 1983). A special medical student waiting list of patients was started which included referrals from the medical, surgical or obstetric and gynaecology teams where students might have seen them being interviewed during psychiatric liaison teaching, which was facilitated by UCH already having a strong tradition of teaching a psychosomatic approach to patients.

Following presentations about the scheme at the European Conference on Psychosomatic Research in 1976, the Psychosomatic Clinic in Heidelberg decided to set up a similar scheme (Sturgeon, 1983). A European Commission grant facilitated a joint project between the two centres to plan meetings, hold workshops with students and compare methods, culminating in Heidelberg University setting up its own scheme. This also stimulated UCH to revisit some of the controversies about its scheme, such as the selection of students, the nature of the supervision groups, and different styles of supervision. Medical students who had previously participated in the scheme were also invited back to the department to report how participation in the scheme had continued to influence their work after qualifying as doctors.

Since then, similar Student Psychotherapy Schemes have been set up in medical schools with varying degrees of success. For some years a scheme was run for a few students in the early 1990s in the Department of Psychotherapy at West Middlesex Hospital in London but ceased as it did not receive sufficient backing from the medical school (West, 2002). Another scheme operated in Oxford for a few years. Similarly, a scheme set up in the Université Vaudois in Lausanne, Switzerland ran for some years until its two supervisors left the department. Other medical schools have allowed students to see patients for shorter periods of supervised psychotherapy than on the UCL Student Psychotherapy Scheme, including a teaching initiative at St. George's Hospital Medical School where all students were involved in a brief (5-week) weekly supervised psychotherapy of one of their patients during their psychiatry clerkship (Crisp, 1986), and since 1995 at the Department of Psychiatry in the University of Toronto in Canada, where medical students take on a patient for 4 months of weekly psychotherapy, while receiving group supervision from a faculty psychiatrist (Shapiro et al., 2009). The latter scheme was modelled after the UCH Student Psychotherapy Scheme and continues to operate today. In the UK, a similar scheme was set up in 1996 for medical students at Bristol University Medical School and continues to successfully operate and develop (see Chapter 4). More recently a Student Psychotherapy Scheme, also specifically modelled on the UCH scheme, has been initiated in the Department of Psychological Medicine in conjunction with the Institute of Psychiatry at King's College London University to enable medical students to see a patient for supervised psychotherapy as an extended Student Selected Component (SSC)[2] for 9 to 12 months (King's College London, 2012). As the scheme grew in popularity some students actually began to choose to study at UCL in order to get on this scheme. By this time, however, demand far outweighed supply, and there were many students who ended up disappointed that they were not allocated to the scheme. Places were limited to 10 to 15 students per year, first by the finite number of supervisors available, and second by the limited number of suitable patients. This led to the introduction of a new process of selecting students by interviewing them, and student Balint groups were eventually offered as an alternative in 2004 (Shoenberg and Suckling, 2004; see Chapter 5) to accommodate the large numbers of students wanting to participate in this scheme.

Remarkably, the scheme has not only survived several mergers and expansions of the medical school, as well as structural iterations of the psychotherapy department in which it is delivered, but remains extremely popular and oversubscribed.

Organisation of the UCL Student Psychotherapy Scheme

The UCL Student Psychotherapy Scheme bridges two separate but linked institutions – a medical school, part of University College London, and a department of psychotherapy, now part of a much larger NHS mental health foundation trust. The functioning of the scheme is therefore not solely confined to those directly involved in its organisation and delivery but also has to take account of its wider institutional settings.

Selection of students

Participation in the scheme is available as an optional educational activity to medical students in their first clinical year when they experience their first significant clinical contact with patients. Because of the scheme's long history, the medical school has always actively supported and promoted it as a worthwhile extra-curricular opportunity available to a minority of medical students. An introductory talk is given at the beginning of the first clinical year, during which we tell the students about the scheme, and also about the student Balint group scheme, their history, aims and practicalities, and what the students might expect to gain from the experience of participating. Students who have recently taken part in the scheme talk about their experience of seeing a patient as a student therapist under supervision, which powerfully conveys the intellectual stimulation, emotional intensity and responsibility that participating in the scheme confers. We then invite all interested students to put their names down if they wish to be interviewed for the scheme. This is in itself a test of their motivation, as many change their mind and decide not to be interviewed. We usually end up interviewing around 40 (out of a total year group of 350) students for the 10 to 15 places available on the scheme each year.

This interview assesses the student's motivation to participate in the scheme and in a rather limited way gauges whether they have any psychological difficulties, such as a depressive illness or eating disorder, that would interfere with doing psychotherapy. We ascertain that students recognise the amount of time (3 to 4 hours per week) involved in making a commitment to doing this scheme and also that they are aware of the responsibility entailed in seeing a patient: the student who expresses anxiety about such a commitment may be more in touch with this than one who appears to be in denial. Previous experience of voluntary work with vulnerable individuals is always an asset. These students will not have had any clinical experience of psychiatry at this stage and we are not testing for prior knowledge of psychiatry, psychology or psychotherapy. We are, however, looking for students who appear enthusiastic, committed and conscientious, and also have some awareness of their limitations and potential vulnerabilities, without appearing too fragile.

Selection of patients

The patients have all been originally referred for psychotherapy by GPs, general psychiatrists or other mental health professionals. They are assessed by a senior member of staff, and after careful consideration of their suitability to see a medical student this is discussed with the patient and their informed consent is obtained. It is explained to the patient that seeing a medical student would offer them an introduction to psychodynamic psychotherapy and that if, after completing the year of treatment, they would like to have further therapy, this can be arranged either in the form of individual or group therapy following another assessment. Although some patients may express a wish to see a qualified and more experienced therapist, surprisingly many are open to seeing a medical student, particularly after a little of the history of the scheme has been explained to them and our experience of how students can be very good therapists. Once the patient agrees, their name is put on the medical student waiting list. The patient, of course, is free to opt out at any time and be given a more experienced therapist. However, in practice, this rarely happens, and most will then start therapy with a student.

Patients with a history of serious self-harm or suicide attempts, serious personality disturbance, drug and alcohol dependence, psychosis or other major mental illness are excluded from seeing a medical student. The patients who tend to do well with students are those with less severe difficulties such as anxiety or minor depression, psychosomatic difficulties, and those with a history of bereavement. Younger patients referred for treatment with chronic depression related to emotional deprivation in childhood, or depressive reactions to physical illnesses also often do well with a student therapist. Younger patients are often more willing to see a student as they find it easier to talk to someone their own age, but students have successfully treated patients of all ages. It is interesting that patients with psychosomatic complaints, who are often thought not to be psychologically minded and therefore resistant to exploratory psychotherapy, seem to do relatively well with medical student therapists (see clinical example in Conclusion). This may be because the students are themselves currently immersed in a medical world focused on the treatment of bodily symptoms and are more able to easily engage than some more experienced psychotherapists with the patient's overt somatic concerns, before gradually being able to help the patient acquire awareness of the underlying psychological meaning and emotional correlates of their symptoms.

One gradual but consistent and significant shift that has occurred in recent years, which has had a negative impact on the ease of finding patients suitable for medical students, has been the increase in the severity of psychopathology typical of the patients referred to the Department of Psychotherapy. This is a reflection of the narrowing of the scope of mental conditions that are funded for treatment within secondary psychiatric services in the NHS, which are now reserved for patients with more serious and enduring mental illnesses and personality disorders, and the expectation that more minor psychiatric and psychological conditions should be treated within a primary care setting. This presents a significant challenge to the organisation of the Student Psychotherapy Scheme in an NHS specialist department within secondary care. Although our experience is that some students under careful supervision may as safely and effectively treat more disturbed patients as junior psychiatrists in training, this may not be the best training experience for the student and issues of clinical risk and patient safety are obviously paramount. One solution may be to encourage GPs and others to specifically refer patients directly for consideration for the scheme and we have periodically written to all local GPs advertising the scheme and explaining which patients might be most suitable. However, the current introduction of 'Payment by Results' to ensure parity of care and cost effectiveness for all mental health services in England may preclude such arrangements as the threshold for referral to secondary services is raised yet further. The financial considerations of supervising students on the scheme are discussed in more detail below.

Selection and role of supervisors

Weekly supervision for the medical students is an essential component of the Student Psychotherapy Scheme. The scheme requires a considerable commitment from its supervisors: not only do they need to dedicate at least 1 hour per week to supervision, but they need to believe in the ethos of the scheme and that student therapists who have no prior qualifications or experience may nevertheless be taught to provide safe and effective treatment for the patient.

Usually our supervisors are medically qualified, as by virtue of this they will have an easier identification with their medical students and be better able to gauge the appropriateness of their reactions and anxieties relative to their specific stage of medical training. Supervising medical student therapists differs from the supervision of postgraduate professionals doing a psychoanalytic or psychotherapy training. The Student Psychotherapy Scheme supervisor must accept that the majority of the students will not have had their own personal therapy, and will have no prior knowledge of psychoanalytic theory or technique. It is therefore important that the supervisor is able to translate psychoanalytic concepts into everyday language and examples, and to avoid formulating complicated hypotheses and interpretations (Becker and Knauss, 1983). The supervisor will also need to accept more limited therapeutic goals for the patient that are feasible in a time-limited treatment by an inexperienced therapist. He or she also needs to be sensitive to the age and developmental stage of the students. Most are in their early twenties and, as such, may not have yet had much exposure to different social or cultural practices or direct experience in the field of personal and sexual relationships, which may become a problem if they feel uncomfortable or unfamiliar with the nature of the patients' difficulties (see below). Students also need some teaching about the varieties of emotional disturbance and of mental illness.

Supervisors should be available, approachable and willing to deal with acute situations or the occasional emergencies that may occur outside the allocated supervision time. It is best if the supervision is done in the department, and that the supervisor is a participating member of the psychotherapy team so that they appreciate the relevant clinical governance issues involved. Sometimes it can be helpful for a senior trainee psychiatrist in psychotherapy to supervise, as their closeness in years to the students may enable them to be sensitive to the students' attitudes and lifestyles. Ultimately, the supervisor carries a dual responsibility both for the patient and the medical student.

Practicalities

Students are allocated, usually in the January of their first clinical year, to a supervision group of three or four students, led by a supervisor, which meets for an hour once a week. To facilitate the students' attendance and ensure that supervisions do not clash with compulsory lectures or clinical work, the supervision meetings are arranged to take place in the Department of Psychotherapy after 5pm on a weekday, or sometimes earlier on Wednesday afternoons, which are allocated by the medical school as free time for students to pursue their own activities. Similarly, students are encouraged to see their patients at 5 or 6pm in the evening, when rooms are more freely available but also to ensure that the students can regularly make and be on time for their sessions. It is essential at an early stage to emphasise to the students the importance of reliability and consistency in psychotherapeutic treatment. This means that they need to arrange to see the patient punctually at the same time on the same day in the same room, which is set up each week in the same manner. These arrangements are facilitated for the students by their supervisor, who can also model reliability and punctuality, but also critically by the administrative staff who are involved in the running of the scheme by virtue of their booking the rooms, as well as appreciating the scheme's ethos and the anxieties of the students. Students also need to be aware before they start on the scheme that they will not take on a patient immediately, which means that their participation in the scheme is likely to extend well into the following academic year when it may become more difficult to see the patient at the same time due to their having to do clinical placements that are further away from central London. Historically, the medical school has been sympathetic to students doing the scheme and has sometimes prioritised their choice of such placements nearer London. Similarly, our consultant colleagues in other medical specialties have allowed students to miss some of their clinical teaching in order to attend supervision or see their patients. However, with an expanding medical school population, increasing demands and expectations of medical students, and an evolving curriculum, the Student Psychotherapy Scheme must adapt and accommodate to continue to survive.

Financial considerations

The scheme was initially run independently in the Department of Psychological Medicine at UCH by psychiatrists employed within that department. Since this psychotherapy service became incorporated into the Camden and Islington Mental Health and Social Care Trust, the scheme has been financially underpinned by 'Service Increment for Teaching' (SIFT) funds, which is money paid by the Department of Health to hospital trusts and general practices to offset the service costs associated with undergraduate medical and dental teaching. SIFT is a component of the multi-professional education and training (MPET) levy, which also comprises postgraduate medical, dental, nursing and allied health professions, and some other clinical specialties. In 2003, the monies generated via this income stream were sufficient to fund an additional two-session consultant psychiatrist in psychotherapy post in the trust specifically to run the Student Psychotherapy Scheme. The trust continues to receive SIFT funds to support the organisation of the scheme and supervision of the students. However, the Department of Health has been engaged in a major policy review of the MPET levy in the last few years, and it is likely that SIFT monies will be reduced with consequent uncertainty regarding the future financial arrangements of the scheme. Although the scheme demands organisational and supervision time from psychotherapists working within the Department of Psychotherapy, the students are also providing a service to the department in seeing some of their patients. This is similar to the arrangement in which honorary trainee psychotherapists see patients without remuneration in return for receiving supervision on their work. In 2013 the scheme became an SSC (Student Selected Component), which has further changed the amount of SIFT money it generates.

Seeing the patient and difficulties encountered

Starting with the patient

When the student starts attending the supervision group he or she will not take on a patient immediately, but will be first encouraged to read some brief basic texts on psychotherapy[3] and, depending on the supervisor, will discuss some of the basic principles of psychotherapy. He or she also spends the first few weeks listening to and learning from the accounts of therapy sessions from students in the year above who are still seeing their patients and attending the supervision group. Although this can make the practical logistics of allocation of students to supervision groups somewhat complicated, the overlapping of students about to start the scheme with those nearing completion is a more effective and powerful method of teaching the practice of psychotherapy than theoretical instruction, as by this means new students hear live examples of clinical material from the patient sessions of their more experienced peers.

The student is encouraged to take on a patient and, depending on the number of patients available on the waiting list, will be given the file of a patient to read (ideally one assessed by the supervisor) and then discuss in supervision. The student is then prepared for the first meeting with the patient by discussing some of the basic boundaries and parameters of the initial therapeutic contact and thinking about possible scenarios that might occur, such as the patient who talks too much or, alternatively, is silent; how to deal with personal questions from the patient such as queries about the student's age or qualifications; or questions about the nature of the treatment. Although supervisors may vary in the degree and detail of preparation they give the student, I try to provide the student with a basic framework of what he or she might say and do in this initial meeting, which will include confirming a regular session time and letting the patient know about the usual psycho-therapy arrangements regarding breaks in therapy. I also insist that the student visit and arrange the room beforehand and think carefully about details such as the arrangement of chairs, where the clock is placed, and how they will introduce themselves and fetch the patient from the waiting room.

Initial anxieties

Most students are understandably anxious about seeing the patient for the first time, and may voice fears that they will not know what to do or that the patient will know that they have no experience and may be disappointed or under-mine them in some way. Although providing a framework in preparation for the initial meeting with the patient may go some way to allay such anxieties, one important aim of the scheme is to enable students to learn to tolerate uncertainty in their interactions with patients and to be aware of the limitations of their knowledge. This requires a shift in style of communication with the patient, away from an 'interrogation mode', which is the main method that students will have been taught, i.e. asking a list of preconceived questions, towards a less structured form of listening. This necessitates a shift in style that is not only in the verbal sphere, but also in the student's behaviour: he or she must now refrain from taking notes in the patient's presence, and must also situate himself or herself at the same level as the patient by sitting in a similar chair next to him or her, rather than at a desk. The removal of these habitual accoutrements of the doctor–patient interaction may make some students feel disempowered and anxious. These students may need time to be able to foster and appreciate the therapeutic potency of a different type of communi-cation – an interpersonal space which is not prestructured by the doctor, but one which is led by the patient and gradually allows for the detection and emergence of information that was not immediately evident in the patient's initial presentation. This is, of course, the realm of non-verbal, emotional and unconscious communications to which both student and patient will gradually be introduced, aided by the support and skill of the supervisor and the containment of the supervision group. Particularly anxious students may be also reassured when they realise that the patient's anxieties about the initial encounter are almost always greater than their own!

Ongoing work

Most students, however, quickly and confidently adjust to their new role as psychotherapists by conscientiously taking in and applying what they are learning in the supervision group. We ask the students to record as much as they can remember of each session as soon as is feasible after the session has finished, also noting the behaviour of the patient, silences, the mood and ambience of the session, and the feelings and thoughts engendered in the student that may not have been verbalised. These written accounts form the raw material of each supervision to be discussed by the supervisor and the other students, and will facilitate the supervisor in gradually introducing the student to the art of psychodynamic listening and the technique of therapeutic practice. This will include teaching some of the basic theoretical principles and concepts of psychoanalytic psychotherapy, such as unconscious processes, the importance of dreams, wishes and fantasies, free association, repression, resistance, projection and other psychological mechanisms of defence, transference and counter-transference, the need for boundaries and for restraint from self-disclosure, and the importance of attachment, dependence and separation in the patient's development, often evident around breaks. However, we also promote the student's freedom to find his or her own style, one which must be informed by theoretical principles but that also feels natural and authentic, and which will facilitate the development of a positive therapeutic alliance with the patient.

Through their encounters with their patients these theoretical concepts quickly acquire meaning and affective resonance. Students are often surprised at the intensity of the experience for both themselves and the patient, how they may find that they spend a significant part of their time away from the patient or supervision thinking, reflecting and even dreaming about the patient; but they are also frequently unprepared for the powerful impact that they have on the patient. Here the concepts of transference and countertransference may become alive, when, for example, the patient, despite having been told that they are medical students, nevertheless pushes them into a position of authority and assumed knowledge, which may give rise to feelings of guilt and inadequacy, or more rarely superiority and omnipotence, in the student, which the supervisor must be sensitive to.

For example, one female student, whose patient was a woman in her sixties who felt trapped in a relationship with her elderly yet domineering mother, was surprised at how rapidly the patient related to the student as a powerful maternal figure despite the large difference in age and generational values. This made the student feel unexpectedly intensely guilty, as well as somewhat irritated, which felt out of proportion in relation to any doubts she had about her lack of experience. The supervisor suggested that perhaps the student was experiencing feelings unconsciously projected by the patient: that the patient was unable to consciously acknowledge her conflictual feelings of anger and guilt towards her mother, but instead behaved in ways which provoked others, in this case the student, to feel them instead. Over the course of the therapy the student was facilitated in gradually interpreting this transferential-countertransferential dynamic to the patient, who was then able to see more clearly how she unconsciously assumed a subservient role towards others that she consciously resented. This enabled her to achieve a better sense of separation from her mother and lessened her fears that she would be left with tremendous guilt after her mother died.

Hearing the other students' accounts of their therapy sessions with their patients in the supervision group is a vital part of each student's learning process. This enables them to see similarities between their patients and others, and to appreciate how emotional needs and conflicts have common sources (Sturgeon, 1983). The 'open' supervision group structure, in which new students overlap with those in the year above, also allows for the former to learn about the different phases of therapy and be better prepared for what might unfold in the treatment of their own patient. The students also implicitly support each other, and their contributions towards each other's cases becomes an essential form of peer supervision. Of course, the role of the supervisor as an experienced psychotherapist is also paramount, and his or her behaviour, such as starting and ending supervision groups on time and relating to the students in a respectful manner, may be very important as a modelling experience at a stage when the students are being exposed to a range of communication styles and sometimes questionable 'bedside manner' in the doctors that they observe. During the hour's supervision there is usually time for two students to present their sessions in detail in a group of four. I usually start each supervision session with a quick update from all of the students to ensure that there is nothing urgent that a student wishes to discuss if it is not their turn to present.

Crises and acting out

The students are encouraged to contact the supervisor if they are worried about anything during or after their session with their patient. Because the students may see their patients on a different day from their supervision group and in the early evening, their own supervisor may not be in the department at that time. However, there is always a senior clinician available in the department should any difficulties arise. For example, one patient who had only recently started therapy with a student refused to leave the room following the end of the session. Eventually one of the supervisors saw the patient and was able to resolve this situation.

Breaks in treatment may be particularly sensitive times for the patient, and cover should be arranged if the student is going to be away for a significant period of time. This could be letting the patient know that they can contact the department and see another therapist if necessary. Usually the student's leave is no longer than a couple of weeks, but this may be much longer over the summer period or if the student decides to extend seeing the treatment well into the following year when there are likely to be more prolonged clinical attachments outside London.

> One gifted student, who was encouraged to continue to see her patient for 18 months as she was thought to be doing well, was offered the opportunity to do a 4-week clinical attachment in a hospital abroad. Although this was agreed by her supervisor, and the patient was told about the break well in advance, with no anticipated problems, the student was surprised and worried when she returned to find that the patient had created a crisis in which she had cut herself and smashed up her flat, warranting input from the community psychiatric team in the student's absence. Although the patient had a history of this type of behaviour, this had not emerged in the treatment until now. While obviously very distressing for all concerned, this was a useful learning experience for the student regarding the power of the transference, and understanding how the patient's feelings of attachment, dependence, abandonment and aggression, which had their roots in the patient's history, were triggered by the student's leave. These were discussed in supervision and the student was able to resume therapy and explore what had happened with the patient.

Although the occurrence of serious clinical incidents such as this have been rare in the history of the Student Psychotherapy Scheme, the supervisor should be alert to the possibility of more minor incidents of acting out between the student and patient. Students may feel pressured by the patient to give them their personal mobile phone number, chat on the way to the therapy room after collection from the waiting room, or even to acquiesce to a patient's request to meet up for a drink between sessions. Understanding that boundaries are necessary in psychotherapy not solely as the arbitrary rules of a treatment approach, or to protect the privacy of the therapist, but because many patients have a history of confused or lack of boundaries which they may re-enact in their therapy, may be helpful for the student.

Lack of progress in the patient

Many of the patients report feeling helped by their student therapists surprisingly quickly, with some showing remarkable symptomatic improvement very rapidly, such as the young woman whose hysterical foot drop disappeared within 2 weeks of starting with a student therapist (Sturgeon, 1983). However, students on the scheme need to be prepared for the slow pace of change of many patients who have psychological difficulties and to understand that the removal of symptoms may not be the cure but only the beginning of therapy, revealing underlying anxieties and personality difficulties that need to be addressed (see essay on students' experiences in Chapter 3 by Elsa Gubert). Students may feel disillusioned when their patient does not seem to be making any progress, or seems to be getting worse. One year is experienced as a significant length of time for most students at this stage of their life as young adults who are still maturing and making significant discoveries and changes. Tolerating psychological stasis in the patient or impasses in treatment may be particularly difficult for students whose own personal and professional trajectories are taking off in exciting directions. Here, the stimulation of hearing about other students' patient's progress in the group supervision may be vital in sustaining the student's interest and commitment to the patient.

Patients who terminate treatment prematurely present a particular challenge for the Student Psychotherapy Scheme. Our experience is that the frequency of drop-out for patients seeing medical students is no higher than other psychotherapy patients receiving treatment from more experienced therapists. Nevertheless, when this occurs it can leave the student feeling demoralised and inadequate, believing that they have done something wrong or that if they were more experienced they would have been able to keep the patient in treatment. It can be helpful if the student can be encouraged to discuss such feelings of failure within the supervision group. These can be linked to a discussion of how doctors may deal with failures of treatment in general, such as the patient dying of cancer or chronic medical conditions that are resistant to treatment, to appreciate how even experienced physicians may feel inadequate or guilty. Some students are willing to take on another patient, but this requires the student to dedicate yet more time to the scheme in the year ahead, which may not be possible due to the demands of their medical studies. However, even if the student does not opt to start with another patient, it is important to encourage them to remain in the supervision group for the remainder of the original allocated time period, not only to continue to learn from hearing the other students' cases, but to work through some of the difficult feelings that they may have been left with by the patient leaving and to avoid re-enacting them like the patient by dropping out of the scheme prematurely.

Personal difficulties of students

The supervisor's role is to foster an atmosphere of trust in which feelings about the patients may be openly discussed, and one of the key functions of the supervision group is to deal with the students' countertransference reactions to their patients when they interfere with the students' therapeutic capacity. Occasionally the patient's difficulties may resonate with unforeseen personal difficulties in the student and trigger unresolved conflicts which may be difficult to handle.

> For example, one patient referred with depression became increasingly dependent and clinging with the student, who found this difficult to tolerate and it resulted in her feeling irritated towards the patient, which made her feel guilty. She was able to discuss these countertransference feelings in supervision and admitted that the patient reminded her of her mother, who had developed multiple sclerosis when the student was a child. It transpired that the feelings evoked by the patient stemmed from unresolved conflicting feelings towards her mother: of anger that she had become an invalid and was unable to look after her like a normal mother, and guilt for feeling this and for avoiding caring for her by escaping into her studies. It was likely that this student had unconsciously chosen to do the scheme to alleviate some of these feelings of guilt by being given the chance to look after another patient.

Very few of the students will have had or are receiving personal psychotherapy, and the supervision group may provide a therapeutic function as students become more aware of their own emotional vulnerabilities through their experience of being with their patients. When the scheme was founded, supervisors were actively encouraged to practice limited therapy of the student where necessary in combination with their supervision (Ball and Wolff, 1963). How supervisors handle any emerging personal difficulties of their students today may vary, but this is clearly a delicate area and supervisors must be sensitive to the student's transferences to them and tread carefully so that the student's problems are not unnecessarily exposed to peers in the group supervision. Recommending that the student seek his or her own personal psychotherapy is sometimes advisable and the supervisor may help the student to find a suitable therapist.

Ending therapy with the patient

As in any time-limited therapy, the ending of the treatment offered should be carefully planned with the patient. Often the patient's original presenting symptoms or complaints may return towards the end of a treatment and students may need reassurance that this does not indicate a failure of the treatment, but represents the unconscious expression of a temporary regression in the patient triggered by feelings of rejection, abandonment and dependence associated with the ending. The students need help with these anxieties and to formulate appropriate interpretations to the patient.

Students are often surprised at how significant they have become to their patient and also how attached they have become to this person as well as to the supervision group and the scheme as a whole, which has become an integral part of their lives for the past year. The feelings evoked at this time of separation for both patient and student will again need careful handling by the supervisor to ensure that appropriate boundaries are maintained and an ending can occur without leaving either party with unmanageable painful feelings. This is often a time when the question of meeting the patient outside therapy arises, and the student may need reminding why this may not be in the patient's best interests, for example, to agree to his or her invitation to 'meet for a drink' after the therapy has ended. The issue of whether or not to accept gifts that the patient may bring in the last session is also relevant, and supervisors will differ in their advice on this. It is sometimes helpful to widen the discussion to exploring the clinical and ethical considerations of the appropriateness of social contact between a doctor and his or her patients in general.

Students may be concerned about the welfare of their patient following termination, particularly if it seems that they could have benefited from a longer therapy. Ideally the question of further treatment for the patient will have been discussed in supervision prior to the ending of the therapy, so that the student can let the patient know that they may be reassessed in the department if they feel that they need further treatment. In practice, many patients feel sufficiently helped by the student and do not wish to continue treatment with anyone else. Some will request further therapy, and ideally will be seen by the person who originally assessed them after 2 or 3 months (unless there is an urgent indication to see them sooner) to allow for a sufficient period of time in which they can reflect on their experience with the student. For some patients further therapy may be thought beneficial, which may be group therapy within the department, or more intensive individual psychotherapy that they may access via a low-fee psychotherapy training scheme.

Following the ending with the patient we ask the student to write a detailed structured report summarising the therapy of their patient to form part of the patient's clinical record. This is a chance for the students to demonstrate their ability to integrate theoretical concepts into their clinical work and to assimilate and consolidate what they have learnt from their experience of participation in the scheme.

Outcomes and future directions

The outcomes of a project may be unexpected and not always predicted from its original aims. The UCL Student Psychotherapy Scheme started with the specific aim of deepening the students' understanding of the doctor–patient relationship via a psychodynamic approach. This remains the primary aim of the scheme and, correspondingly, the expected outcomes in the students who have completed the scheme might be an increased understanding of the psychodynamic aspects of the doctor–patient relationship and an enhanced capacity to relate to their patients. This might include, in no particular order:

- being able to adopt a less structured interview style in which a special type of listening discerns non-verbal and less conscious communications that underpin and sustain the patient's disease;
- appreciating how the patient's history of attachment may influence his or her compliance with treatment;
- tolerating confusion, uncertainty, silences, emotional distress and lack of therapeutic progress;
- acknowledging the emotional impact on the student/doctor of patients and how understanding these emotional reactions may enhance diagnosis and management of the patient's illness;
- recognising the defence mechanisms utilised by the patient and their contribution to the course of their illness;
- discerning the attitudes and roles that the patient unconsciously attributes to the doctor;
- appreciation of the need to maintain appropriate professional boundaries;
- increasing the student's capacity for psychological mindedness and empathy;
- promoting a 'whole person' approach to medicine.

Our own experience is that students do develop at least some of these skills as they progress through the scheme and the few published papers by students about their experiences of the scheme would appear to confirm this (Garner, 1981; Garner et al., 1985; Clifford, 1986; Hoy, 2002; Antonelou, 2010). This is explored further in Chapter 3. However, more objective methods than these anecdotal reports are needed to define, realise and evidence such teaching objectives in order to persuade medical schools that such a labour-intensive teaching initiative only available to a minority of the overall medical student population is a worthwhile endeavour. As the teaching of communication skills has become more central in the medical student curriculum, there is increasing interest in which teaching methods most effectively enable medical students to translate intellectual knowledge of communication styles into enduring interpersonal and emotional skills that will enhance their future relationships with patients. Chapter 8 will examine in more detail how we have attempted to empirically research the scheme to measure its impact on the students and whether some of these outcomes can be achieved.

One unexpected outcome of our research was discovering that participation in the scheme influenced students' choice of career, in that students who did the scheme with no prior interest in becoming a psychiatrist were significantly more likely to choose psychiatry as a career following qualification than students who did not participate in the scheme. A further significant outcome of this study was to discover that many of the participants who did not become psychiatrists reported that the scheme had been a very positive experience and relevant to their later clinical work as GPs or hospital specialists, enabling them to listen and communicate better with their patients (Yakeley et al., 2004). The scheme's experiential method of learning and the experience of having prolonged contact with a patient were two factors that many students felt were most valuable as a learning experience for their later practice as doctors.

Our interest in elucidating the significant outcomes of the scheme should not, of course, be limited to those related to the participating medical students, but must include the experiences and outcomes of the participating patients. Chapter 8 also describes the research to back our clinical experience that the majority of patients do well with a student therapist, achieving as good, if not better, outcomes for the patient as postgraduate core trainees in psychiatry who are obliged to see a psychotherapy case as a mandatory part of their training.

The most significant and overarching outcome, however, which its founders may not have predicted, is the scheme's extraordinary longevity: it continues to operate and develop after more than half a century and remains extremely popular. It has not only weathered many local changes in both the medical school and Department of Psychotherapy from which it is delivered, but continues to flourish despite wider changes in medical education, as well as the relative decline in the acceptance of the psychodynamic psychotherapy approach compared to the cognitive-behavioural paradigm within the National Health Service. Although the scheme continues to face significant challenges, such as the new MBBS curriculum at UCL Medical School as well as changes in commissioning arrangements for patients nationally, the dedication and enthusiasm of its participating teachers, students and patients will ensure that the UCL Student Psychotherapy Scheme continues to survive and inspire other medical schools to develop similar schemes.

To conclude with the words of one participating student:

> My perspective of medicine has changed. I no longer feel compelled to search for quick-fix remedies for physical ills. I have learned to approach patients holistically and to appreciate the power of communication in healing. I believe that the skills learned will have an impact on my whole career.
>
> (Hoy, 2002, p. 57)

Notes

1   The Student Psychotherapy Scheme (SPS) was originally initiated in the Outpatient Department of Psychological Medicine in University College Hospital (UCH), London for medical students at University College Hospital Medical School. In 1987 Middlesex Hospital and University College Hospital merged their

medical schools to form University College & Middlesex School of Medicine (UCMSM). Shortly after this the UCH Department of Psychological Medicine merged with the Psychotherapy Department of the Middlesex Hospital to form the UCH Department of Psychotherapy. In 1998, UCMSM merged with the Royal Free Medical School, to form the Royal Free & University College Medical School, which in 2008, was officially renamed UCL Medical School. In 2000 the Department of Psychotherapy became part of Camden and Islington Mental Health and Social Care Trust, but continued to be based in the Outpatient Department at UCH, now part of the University College London Hospitals (UCLH) Trust. The UCH Department of Psychotherapy merged with the Royal Free Department of Psychotherapy and moved to its current location in King's Cross to become the Camden Psychodynamic Psychotherapy Service in Camden and Islington Foundation Trust in 2008.

2   Student Selected Components are optional modules within the undergraduate medical syllabus in UK medical schools introduced in 2002 following the recommendations of the General Medical Council (GMC) that the syllabus should include student choice.

3   *Introduction to Psychotherapy*, by Bateman, Brown and Pedder (2010), first published in 1979 and now in its fourth edition, published by Routledge, remains an excellent introductory text for students of psychotherapy.

Chapter 2

Experiences of supervisors on the UCL Student Psychotherapy Scheme

Christine Van Duuren and Jennifer Johns

LEARNING THROUGH EXPERIENCING

Christine Van Duuren

> Education is not the filling of a pail, but the lighting of a fire.
> Attributed to W.B. Yeats (1865–1939)

Yeats eloquently sums up the essence of a lively educational experience which is so true of what our Student Psychotherapy Scheme aims to be by providing a real-life setting in which creative learning can take place. This is a personal account of my experiences as a supervisor on this scheme.

The main aim of our scheme is to help students improve their capacity to relate to patients by learning about a psychoanalytic approach to psychotherapy. Naturally we are very much aware of the need for the patients to benefit from their psychotherapeutic experience too.

During their selection interview many students express regret at the fact that they have little opportunity to become acquainted with patients at a deeper level. Usually they want to take part in this scheme because it offers an opportunity to engage in an ongoing relationship with a patient over a prolonged period of time. Some may have in mind a future specialisation in psychiatry or psychotherapy but there is no expectation on our part that participating students will choose this career path.

> One student said that he wanted to become a brain surgeon. 'I want to fix people', he said, with a degree of self-irony. From the start, however, he recognised that the approach of psychotherapy offered valuable benefits and was aware of the need to adapt to its more reflective outlook. In the supervision group he was willing to think about the relative merits of different interpersonal approaches. Like many other students, at the end of the year he felt that his communication skills had greatly improved.

Students are more open minded and less rigid about learning new theories and ways of communicating than trainee psychiatrists, so at this early stage in their career they are in a favourable position to take advantage of this learning opportunity. However, this is not an easy option for the students and it is part of the interviewing and selection process to warn them of the degree of commitment required. They will need to invest a significant amount of their time and energy for more than a year, seeing a patient, writing detailed process notes and attending the weekly supervisions. Participating in the scheme also requires a large emotional investment on the part of the students. Until last year the students did not get any official recognition for their efforts, but now our scheme is offered as a Student Selected Component (SSC) by the medical school.

For us, being supervisors is not an easy task either. We feel passionate about our teaching role but are also very much concerned with the welfare and safety of the patients. We are exposing patients to a situation in which their psychological well-being is in the hands of someone with little experience. As supervisors we feel very responsible in our involvement, guiding and nurturing the students and encouraging best practice. A careful balance needs to be struck between the different relationships that are at play, which requires subtle management. Naturally, supervisors need to approach the students sensitively, and intermittently we have to cope with our concern about unexpected developments that may occur in the therapies conducted by the students.

> Ms C was a middle-aged woman who had suffered considerably in her early life, leaving her rather fragile as an adult. She struggled with relationships and had given up activities that had offered her some satisfaction. After a somewhat difficult start in the therapy with a medical student, she settled down in this therapy, which she came to value. However, she suffered several serious adverse events in quick succession. This was more than Ms C could cope with and she became very depressed. She isolated herself at home and stopped coming to her sessions. Both the student-therapist and the supervisor worried a great deal about her deteriorating mental state and the associated risk. The supervisor discussed these concerns with team members and with Ms C's GP. The student maintained telephone contact with the patient. To everyone's relief, after some weeks Ms C became able to respond to the student's sensitive approaches and resumed her sessions.

The students value the opportunity to build an in-depth relationship with a patient. Moreover, in the course of the psychotherapeutic work with the patients they acquire a great deal of knowledge and experience, both about communication and about psychological processes. The patients benefit as they can be seen sooner than others on longer waiting lists and are seen by dedicated and sensitive people. From the supervisors' point of view, this work with the students is a satisfying experience, notwithstanding the heavy responsibility that they take on. Supervisors enjoy observing the students' relationships with their patients evolving and seeing how these students develop. Finally, there is benefit for the department, in that it means that more patients can be taken into treatment.

Improving communication

Listening is a very important skill in any setting and so is the need to be open and receptive. In psychotherapy listening happens at a deeper level. One much quoted paper (Bunting et al., 1998) revealed that doctors who interrupt their patients early are more likely to have a complaint made against them. Another study revealed that interrupting early can lead to some symptoms not being elicited in the consultation (Beckman and Frankel, 1984). Our students are at a stage in their training in which they are learning to adopt a more directive stance. We need to help them understand the limitations of this customary approach and to explore other options. This is particularly important in the psychotherapy setting, where the aim is to elicit information that the patient is barely or not at all aware of.

> One of the patients was quite an anxious young woman who had done reasonably well in life in that she had a job and she had friends. Her reason for seeking therapy was her low mood and her difficulty in establishing lasting relationships with men. She had experienced a traumatic upbring-ing and coped mostly by denying her emotional difficulties. The student was a kind-hearted, down-to-earth woman. During the early phase of the therapy the patient became more aware of her dissatisfaction with her past and present life. In response to this she reinforced her defences. The student was puzzled. Her own rational approach to life made it difficult for her to understand the convoluted way in which the patient tried to establish an internal equilibrium. She genuinely wanted to understand the patient and tried to achieve this by asking more and more questions. The patient felt threatened and put on the spot. She was as puzzled as the student, she was unable to answer the questions and felt misunderstood, an experience she had had throughout her life. It took a lot of careful work in supervision to help the student understand that the patient required a more reflective interaction that would allow space in which understanding might emerge.

It is equally natural to want to offer advice to someone in trouble, and to try and solve their problems. Although our students are usually already aware of the fact that this is not what we do in psychotherapy, old habits die hard. Their wish to alleviate distress makes it difficult for them to refrain from active intervention. The student-therapist creates the space in which discoveries can be made and understanding can be developed, eventually bringing relief for the patient. The supervision groups offer a great opportunity to help the students to question their habitual way of interacting and engaging with patients, to relinquish a more traditional authoritative or 'knowing' stance, and to reflect on whether this furthers or hinders communication.

Although students learn the basic concepts of psychoanalytic psychotherapy and how to apply them, their theoretical knowledge is limited at the start and only increases to a certain extent. In spite of these limitations students and patients will develop an understanding of the impact of the past on the present and insight into the unconscious conflicts underlying the patients' difficulties. Many therapeutic factors are not contingent on theoretical knowledge. For the patient it is very important to tell their story and be listened to by someone who can identify with them and allow them to safely express their emotions. Such experiences are helpful in doctor–patient relationships in any setting.

> While the student who wished to become a brain surgeon was in theory entirely willing to refrain from 'fixing the patient', in practice he found it difficult to abandon a directive approach. This was encouraged by his patient, who came from an ethnic group where authority figures are imbued with a lot of power. For some time the psychotherapy was a mixture of a psychodynamic and a directive approach. The patient began to say all the right things. The student had learned enough theory to know that this progress might be a further manifestation of the patient's wish to please and this enabled him to listen more carefully and so be more aware of the patient's needs. He could then also gently point out to the patient her compulsion to conform and to help her challenge this. This approach paid off and at the end of the therapy we came to the conclusion that the patient had become more insightful and had also improved.

Selection of students and patients

At the start there is a careful selection of the students. Students who apply for the scheme are highly motivated and already very much aware of the importance of the relationship between doctor and patient. Therefore they are keen to hone their skills in this respect. All students who express an interest are interviewed by senior therapists in the department. It is a highly competitive process, since there are many more applicants than there are places on the scheme and we find that the great majority of the applicants are very bright and motivated. From the applicants we select those who are particularly sensitive, caring and psychologically minded. They also need to have the strength of character and the commitment to cope with all the demands. A number will have done voluntary work in mental health settings but this is not essential. In terms of their plans regarding future specialisation, this varies greatly. Some are already interested in a career in mental health but most want the experience in order to improve their ability to communicate with their patients and to understand psychological processes associated with any health problems.

The selection of suitable patients is as important as the selection of students. In addition to the normal assessment to determine whether psychotherapy is the approach of choice, we need to find patients who will not test the students excessively. This does not just apply to the severity of the symptoms. In addition we need to identify those patients who have at least some capacity to establish a relationship with their therapist, who can make a commitment to the process and who are unlikely to act out their difficulties in damaging ways. This is one of the stumbling blocks in the scheme. It can be a difficult task to find suitable patients, since patients referred to our psychotherapy department increasingly display significant pathology and are likely to pose major challenges to their therapist. In addition, it is not always possible to recognise hidden pathology during the initial assessment, so unfortunately some of our students are faced with challenging patients.

The supervision groups

Each supervisor is responsible for a group of three or four students. The new students join students who have been in the group since the previous year and who already have a patient in treatment. These more experienced students will tell the new recruits about their psychotherapeutic work. This enables the new students to familiarise themselves with the work of the older student group, including the way they conduct sessions, and how they reflect on and discuss clinical material in the supervision group. The older students are in the later stages of the year of therapy and have developed an understanding of their patients and the psychotherapeutic process. The new members of the group learn through listening and are also encouraged to participate in the discussions.

It is heartening to see the new students' enthusiasm. We need to gently guide them and help them contain their emotions. Their compassion, empathy and intuition are already apparent at this early stage. After a short while I offer two or three tutorials, not only to impart knowledge, but also to provide an opportunity to attend to students' emotions and anxieties. The fundamental principles of psychotherapy are discussed including basic theoretical concepts such as the unconscious, transference and countertransference, as well technical issues such as the method of free association and interpretation. I like to demonstrate these processes by looking at daily interactions. In discussions about the unconscious and its manifestations, students soon find examples in their own lives and those of the people around them. This is the first step in helping them to listen with 'a third ear' (Reik, 1948).

As supervisors we also help students to understand the links between past and present in people's, and therefore their patients' lives. Students are encouraged to think about the patients' current object relations in the light of their past experiences. We help them to recognise the complexity of the connections so as to help them build a narrative together with the patient, to recognise patterns and create a sense of continuity.

One student realised that his patient, Mr D, had a tendency to seek out father figures in his life but that according to this student 'the role models he selected had seemingly flawed characters and all ended up hurting or disappointing him in some way'. Mr D 'sought out environments where the terms were dictated by some enigmatic authority over whom he had no control and whom he had to abide by'. The student linked Mr D's attitude to the fact that his father had left the family when he was very young, an event over which he had been powerless but which had had devastating consequences for him. A theme of unfairness cropped up several times during the therapy, 'as did the idea that his fate was determined by some unknowable outside force that was controlling his destiny'. In the transference the student noted that Mr D saw him as an authority figure, who, like his father, could have the power to let him down. In response Mr D felt compelled to deny his need for the therapist and to try and reverse their roles. While this offered a temporary relief, ultimately the consequences of this defensive manoeuvre were detrimental to the patient. The turning point in the therapy came when the student was able to demonstrate to the patient how his attitude interfered with the progress in the therapy. Since the student conveyed this in an empathic way, the message came across and the relationship deepened for the rest of the therapy.

The importance of the relationship between patient and student therapist needs to be discussed in supervision. Students already understand the need for rapport and for a therapeutic alliance; however, we help them to become acquainted with the nature of a relationship as it develops within the psychoanalytic model, since this may be somewhat different from the type of relationship they have been used to, both professionally and personally. Students are very much aware of the responsibility they are taking, but it is hard for them to anticipate what an intense and sometimes complex role they will come to play in the lives of some patients. We also need to help the students understand that they need to give the patient their full attention, to be non-judgemental and to use their intuition and empathy. They will be aware of the importance of creating a space in which the patient can express their emotions.

Consistency in the therapeutic setting is vital and students quickly learn about the importance of being reliably there for their patient and that of telling them well in advance about any forthcoming breaks in the therapy, as well as the importance of being consistent emotionally.

Sometimes students have preconceptions about psychotherapy, for example, that the therapist should be a 'blank screen' and they may wonder how much they are allowed to smile, or how to respond to the patient's emotions. One student thought that therapists should never break a silence. Another asked if you should apologise if the patient gets upset. This latter question is not just a question about the rules of the interaction, but it also suggests unease with the patient's emotions. This student needed to learn the difference between creating a space for the patient to express their emotions and being responsible for inflicting pain.

I like to foster a spirit of openness and creativity in the tutorials and supervisions. Some students may be sceptical about the psychodynamic approach and it is important to allow them to voice their doubts and respond to them seriously. It is satisfying to see a student's face light up when a concept is beginning to make sense, perhaps weeks after it was originally discussed.

> A student had read about the Oedipus complex and brought this up in a tutorial group. She wondered if this was still considered a valid concept in our work. As she asked the question, a certain unease was apparent in her demeanour. Naturally, for someone who was new to the ideas of psychoanalysis, the concept does not make immediate sense. I told the group that in the literature there are certain dissenting voices with respect to the validity of the Oedipus complex but that I myself felt it to be very helpful in understanding patients. I gave some examples of my own practice. More importantly, during the supervision session that followed, dynamics to do with triangulation and exclusion could be clearly detected in the clinical material under discussion. I explained the link between these manifestations and the Oedipus complex. This provided a lively illustration to the original theoretical question.

Some months after joining the group the student will be allocated a patient. The supervisor and the group together read the available clinical information about each of the pre-selected patients. The supervisor will by then know the group sufficiently to form an opinion about the individual students. This will guide decisions about arranging suitable pairings of students with patients.

> One female patient had had a lot of bad experiences with men, including sexual abuse. The group wondered whether she might be better seen by a female therapist. On the other hand it was thought that it might be beneficial for the patient to be offered the opportunity to have a good experience with a man, different from her previous experiences. One of the male students was particularly keen to take her on and the supervisor agreed. This turned out to be a good decision.

The first psychotherapy session

Now it is time for the first meeting with the patient. The students are not fully prepared but they will have discussed many issues in tutorials and supervision, such as how to introduce themselves to their patient, whether to shake the patient's hand, whether they may smile and what they can safely disclose about themselves to their patient. Many students will feel somewhat apologetic, feeling that they are only students after all. The group discussions help them to find a position that they feel relatively comfortable with.

The first session with the new patient is a source of many emotions, mostly a combination of excitement and anxiety. Enthusiasm and optimism may need to be tempered by the supervisor, and anxiety alleviated. Students will have been prepared for any anxiety-provoking situations that may occur in the early sessions. One example of this is the possibility of silences, which can create discomfort in both student and patient. The need to get it 'right' can put pressure on the student, which in turn can be inhibiting and create a tension in the student–patient relationship. Therefore, I seek to facilitate an approach in the students that is natural to them rather than risk them feeling hampered by a sense of how it should be done. Adjustments can be made over time.

Immediately after each session the student writes a process recording, as accurately as they remember it. They are encouraged to also note the feelings the patient expresses, as well as what they experience themselves. This account is then presented at the next supervision group. An open discussion of the material is encouraged, with everybody bringing their ideas. This will promote the type of open-minded receptive listening that we are looking for in therapy. Moreover, it will bring the concepts of transference and particularly counter-transference to life.

We need to keep in mind the students' lack of experience and the need to contain their insecurities. A balance must be struck between open discussion and the provision of specific guidance and advice, for instance, about how to further a path of enquiry or to deal with a challenging situation. At appropriate times we may suggest to the students a particular way of formulating an insight to their patient. This provides a concrete level of support that can increase the students' confidence during the session.

The supervisor seeks to model the type of relationship he or she wants to nurture in the student. Just as it is important for the students to be open minded about the patients, it is important for the supervisor to be open minded about the students. The aim is to promote understanding, which in turn feeds into compassion. There are many parallels. As the learning process is facilitated in supervision, so it is in the session with the patient. As the anxiety in the student is alleviated, so it is for the patient. Similarly, we need to show that we can be robust in handling difficult situations in the supervision setting. This way we can help students to develop an understanding about how to deal both with negative transference and with idealisation by the patient.

Challenges

At times we may be concerned about the way a student has handled a situation. For instance some time into the therapy a student let a colleague know in passing that he had been taking notes during the sessions. The colleague had not thought to bring this up in the tutorials since to her it was self-evident that this is not done. It was important to rectify the situation without the student feeling that he had made a serious mistake. A similar issue applies to time keeping. If the patient is late, the student might decide to add the time on at the end. To them, if they are available, then why not? I like to refrain from the notion of 'rules' and instead encourage the students to think through these issues and to use them as valuable opportunities to further their understanding of both the patient and the psychodynamic process.

As supervisors we are protective of the patients as well as the students. This means that a careful judgement needs to be made about the needs of each. At times this can lead to potentially awkward situations.

> One patient developed a resistant and condescending transference towards his student-therapist. I was worried because I did not know whether the situation could be contained. The patient told the student with some glee how as a child he had got the better of a classmate by peeing on him. I realised that this was a reflection of the patient's stance in relation to the student but was not sure if imparting this knowledge to the group would feel alien and make the student uneasy. In the end I did, to much wonder in the group. The student did not use the insight explicitly in the sessions but the greater understanding he had achieved in contemplating the metaphor lifted some of the pressure he had felt with the patient, making him more solid and free. The laughter in the group also helped to diffuse the tension.

> Another patient developed an erotic transference towards her male therapist. Her interactions became highly flirtatious and she made attempts to change the therapeutic relationship into a more personal one. The student squirmed as he reported his sessions in supervision. Again, respectful humour in the group provided some relief in this difficult situation. The student learned how to maintain his stance as a therapist, without either shaming or encouraging the patient, and over time the behaviour subsided.

The emotional commitment can be particularly challenging. Patients in psychotherapy are encouraged to bring any concerns, feelings and memories to the session and that can test the student's capacity to cope.

> One extreme example of this occurred when a patient's anger was not contained and he threw a tissue box at the wall. Fortunately the student was able to control her shock and became quite firm in response. Subsequently patient and student were able to work together in an effort at understanding the patient's anger.

> Another patient told the student about extreme abuse she had been exposed to as a child, which she had only partially disclosed in the

assessment. The student dealt with the shocking material remarkably well, but for the patient the memories brought on unbearable emotions and she stopped attending. Not only was this unfortunate for the patient, it was also a great disappointment for this very dedicated student. This example also highlights the pitfalls that can occur at the assessment stage.

For students, a patient's negative transference can be hard to bear. Most of them have embarked on a career in medicine because they want to heal and this is an important part of their self-image. When a patient develops a more negative view of the student's ability to provide what the patient is looking for, or perhaps does not recognise their dedication and willingness to help, this can make the student feel hurt. Throughout the process decisions must be made about how much to allow negative transference to develop. Connected with this is the need to develop a view about the degree to which we let the student adopt the role of a friend or confidant to the patient.

One patient had agreed to take part in the scheme but subsequently had become angry about it. In his therapy he expressed a chronic dissatisfaction with what the student contributed and gave him little opportunity to offer something substantial, thereby both conveying and reinforcing his dissatisfaction. Through supervision the student learned to recognise the link between the patient's current presentation and unresolved issues from the past. While this helped him put the uncomfortable situation into perspective, the patient's attitude led to a difficult countertransference experience, which he was very sensitively in touch with. In the supervision he talked about his uneasy feeling of needing to prove something to the patient, to give him some magic piece of advice in order to convince him of his worth and good intentions. The student asked himself painful questions about whether the patient would have done better with a different therapist. Or perhaps, he mused, was he always destined to fail the patient, as so many before him had, friends and relatives as well as professionals. In the supervision an understanding developed of the underlying dynamics within the patient and how these were re-enacted in the transference relationship.

While this was a difficult experience for the student, it was also educational. Any doctor will come into contact with dissatisfied patients. It is then always important to ask oneself honestly whether this is justified under the circumstances or whether this is a result of the patient's internal dynamics. Awareness in the doctor will help prevent either a defensive response to a complaining patient or an unduly accommodating one.

It can also be difficult for students to understand how important they may become in the internal world of the patient.

In one example the student was virtually the only important person in the patient's life and the patient developed a marked attachment to him. Towards the end of the therapy the patient began to make comments minimising the importance of the therapy. The student was ready to accept this at face value, even though this was somewhat disappointing to him. In the supervision group, however, it gradually became clear that the patient's stance was aimed at protecting herself from the pain of ending. Following guidance from the supervisor the group took it upon themselves to look at subsequent sessions and to identify the hidden expressions of distress. They found many. This enabled the student to reappraise the situation and to support the patient more effectively in coming to terms with the ending.

When the outcome is less favourable, this can be difficult for patient and student and a concern for the supervisor. The supervisor always needs to be aware of the importance of supporting students when they feel that they are failing. Some problems can be resolved, in which case it is beneficial for both the patient and the student, but some will lead to the patient dropping out.

A patient was referred for psychotherapy to help her come to terms with a very painful family issue that occurred in the past. The mental turmoil, a large component of which was guilt, had interfered with her well-being over many years. In spite of the student's very sensitive and non-judgemental approach to the patient, the latter became overwhelmed by feelings of guilt and regret, and left the therapy prematurely. In this case the assessor had thought that the difficulties of the patient were external and historical and that she therefore simply needed help in mourning. As the treatment unfolded the problem turned out to be more complex.

Changes in patients and students

As with all therapies, different relationships develop between therapist and patient, depending on the varying characteristics of both. Sometimes a close bond develops, which involves warmth, trust and an ongoing sense of cooperation. This leaves the patient with a sense that something good was offered, which they were able to receive and take away for the future. At other times the therapy has become more of a struggle, but if the difficulties are overcome, both patient and student are left with a sense of achievement about having weathered the storm and a belief that adversities in relationships can be worked through. Either way there will be increased insight and an improved knowledge of where and how things had gone right or wrong in the patient's internal world. Patients will internalise their experience and draw on it in the future.

Examples of practical gains may be the ability to complete a course and take an exam, join a gym, and a reduced need for drugs and casual sex, to name but a few. In terms of relationships, patients have reported getting on better with parents, other relatives and friends.

> One patient reported that his mother had reciprocated his overtures by acknowledging that 'I f****d you up when you were a child'. This in turn helped the patient move on.

Some patients start new relationships. In others there is evidence of a greater capacity for concern, a greater sense of self-awareness or increased assertiveness.

> The patient who in his anger had thrown the box of tissues at the wall said that the therapy had given him time to reflect on his life, which had helped him to accept his past and the possibilities of the future. He felt he could judge situations better and act upon them in a more mature manner.

If a patient discontinues his or her therapy he or she may be offered a review which may result in the offer of further therapy with a more experienced psychotherapist.

Many students tell us about the profound impact the experience has had on them as people and as clinicians. They make it clear how much they have gained in confidence in their dealings with patients on the wards. The skills they have acquired provide them with an increased capacity to understand their patients as whole human beings, with all their emotions. They report an increased capacity to understand them and respond to them. The student who had originally told me that he planned to become a brain surgeon wrote:

> Ms A will always be a special patient to me. The memories of the sessions we spent together may fade with time, but the lessons learnt will not. Since my time with Ms A, I always try and make time for the patients I see. I try to be courteous to them all and think about what I say to them and how they may respond. . . . What I have observed is that patients trust you so much more with such an approach, often saving the time that more abrupt clinicians hope to achieve by skimping on the human side of medicine. . . . Patients trust us with intimate secrets when they come to seek our help, especially so in the case of Ms A. I have slowly begun to understand the gravity of this trust and it has humbled me. I hope that even if I become a high-flying consultant one day that these lessons will keep me grounded and I will not forget that I am there to help the patients and they are not there to help further my career.

Another example describes a more problematic relationship, which had helped the student understand that the avoidance of difficult interactions is not always beneficial. After completing the year of therapy with a somatising patient, she put her learning in the following words:

[Our relationship] became dominated by Ms B's absence from sessions, often without prior cancellation. Towards the end of our sessions together, I began to realise that my desire to help and care about her was becoming a hindrance to her progress, as I could be very non-questioning of her absences, telling her that 'it's alright, at least you made it today'. In retrospect this may have been due to anxieties and insecurities I had about being a medical student; could the cause of her absence be my inexperience, having said the wrong thing at times, or having responded to her discourse in the wrong way? Ultimately it was not helpful to her, as I was validating a safety net she had grown used to using in her adult life: that of her physical illness being an explanation and a get-out clause for other responsibilities relating to herself, her friends and her family.

If the therapy is not brought to a positive end, supervisors will not only be there to support the student with their difficult experience but they will also try and turn the situation into a learning experience. Fortunately, this only happens in a minority of cases.

Conclusion

One patient described his experience of his psychotherapy with his student as 'one of the best decisions I have ever made'. This touches on the heart of our endeavour, which is our wish to provide an enriching experience for patients and students alike. We hope to have lit a fire that will continue to burn in us all for a long time to come. Moreover, in their future career students will hopefully pass on to their colleagues the ethos and the skills that they have acquired by being part of the Student Psychotherapy Scheme.

THOUGHTS ON BEING A SUPERVISOR

Jennifer Johns

For 14 years I was part of the Student Psychotherapy Scheme as a supervisor in the original Department of Psychotherapy at University College Hospital (UCH). When I retired, Christine Van Duuren took over my part in the scheme. As she states, each student, each patient, and each student–patient pairing is different, and this is part of what makes this experience of supervision both fascinating and absorbing for the supervisor. I found that the supervision sessions with the medical students were the part of my working week to which I looked forward the most, and to which I looked back with the most satisfaction. This is not to say that it was in any way simple or free from anxiety, either for the students, the patients or me.

Two opposing points of view come to mind. One is a remark reported to me by one of the students in my group. On a social occasion in her parents' house she told one of their psychotherapist friends that she was seeing a patient under the Student Psychotherapy Scheme. The psychotherapist was horrified that psychotherapy patients were being seen by medical students, and the student was told emphatically that the scheme was dangerous and should not be allowed. My student was very anxious about this, and it took some time and encouragement, including that from the rest of the group, to settle the anxiety down.

The other point of view was expressed at a dinner party where I met two other older doctors, one an academic in a research department, and his spouse, a senior clinician in a non-psychiatric speciality. The warm smiles that spread over each of their faces when I said that I supervised on the scheme were memorable and each told me quite spontaneously that the scheme had been the most rewarding part of their training at UCH in the now-distant past. They had been sorry for those students who had not had this experience, and each said that their capacity to make good relationships with patients and also with colleagues had been enhanced by the scheme.

There is a long and complex journey between these two positions. I can quite understand the concern of the psychotherapist, who had presumably spent many postgraduate years in training for the role, that someone who appeared much too young and inexperienced, only a few years out of school, should be approaching the same task. What the psychotherapist cannot have known about is the careful selection process described by Van Duuren: first the self-selection that brings the students to the initial large meeting where the scheme, its purpose, something of its history, the commitment involved, the drawbacks and the possible rewards are explained; and then the individual interviews to discuss in more detail and in privacy something of each student's own motives, fears and hopes for joining the scheme. This is done to make as sure as possible that the student is well motivated without being idealistic, has at some level an awareness of unconscious processes, even without the sophistication of having studied them, and has enough psychological strength to cope with difficult and sometimes disappointing situations. That a good proportion of the students selected already have experience in carefully listening to people in distress might also be surprising – one young woman whom I supervised had organised a peer-led student counselling service in the college she had attended prior to medical school, several students had worked voluntarily in hostels and hospices, and almost all had completed intercalated degrees, often in psychology, as part of their medical studies. A few were mature students, with life experience, and some had suffered and survived personal losses. In making the selections the students' thoughtfulness and an awareness of the need for commitment to the patients were important. Often the students expressed their concern lest they were not good enough, or anxiety should they have to let the patient down. They were aware, for instance, that the medical school might require them to attend periods of study some distance away from London, and that they might have to miss some sessions. Many were unsure whether they were ready for 'real' responsibility, others were keen for it.

There is a third point in the selection process for those who have been chosen: it happens informally. The selected students are asked to join an already existing group of students for the last few months before the older ones stop seeing their patients and before the newer ones have taken a patient on, to listen and observe, hearing something of the way that those only slightly older have managed. It is an interesting stage for both groups – the older, hearing the anxieties of the newcomers, can recognise how far they have come themselves, and in their wish to help the new arrivals often put things into words that reinforce their own learning, are helpful to the newcomers, and also demonstrate to the supervisor how much they have taken in or discovered for themselves.

It is at this stage that a student who has been despondent that their own hopes for the patient has failed to materialise, and perhaps is facing the patient's own disappointment in the form of anger or withdrawal, can, in recalling the original clinical state, recognise that change has indeed occurred, and that their efforts may not have been in vain. The newer ones can be impressed by their older peers, but also reassured that this difficult task can be undertaken safely, and also that while progress can often be made, it may be slow but is still worthwhile. For the supervisor, watching the interaction between those only slightly more sophisticated and the keen but naive beginners can also be a learning experience. It can leave the supervisor both surprised and full of respect for the future doctors who take their role so seriously. It is now that the supervisor can explain to the newcomers that so far they are not completely committed to the scheme – the important commitment comes with the actual selection of a patient to see, and the act of the initial interview, following which any decision to pull out could have serious consequences for the patient, especially if there is a history of previous rejection. The need for reliability will also have become clear. In my experience, the few students who pulled out at this stage did so because they realised that they couldn't actually make such a commitment to seeing a patient each week for a year.

By the time the student is faced with this final choice, the stories that they have heard from the previous group, and the changes they have heard about, more often than not confirm for them that this is a task worth doing, and they are keen to get on with it. They will have already had guidance about the importance of reliability and boundaries from the older members of the group who also may have spoken of the times that they have been surprised, pleased or put out by their patients, and how they have dealt with that, and of the attitude of the psychotherapist towards the work. Selection of patients for the scheme is another delicate matter, and one in which the supervisors are closely concerned, since they also assess patients referred for psychotherapy, and may well have either seen the prospective patients themselves or have attended the professional meetings at which assessments are discussed and at which decisions are made about the best way forward for individual patients. The selection of patients for individual students is also one to be thought about carefully. The supervisor will try, so far as is possible, to 'match' the pair according to what is known about each participant in the process. Age, gender, ethnicity, even perceptions of social background may be taken into consideration, as well as personality factors.

> One student who supplemented her income by evening work in a small shop decided not to take on a very suitable-sounding patient when she recognised the patient's address as being in the block of flats above the shop, since she was concerned about meeting the prospective patient while in another role herself and losing some of the anonymity that she recognised would be useful to her in her 'new' role.

> Another, who spoke at the first interview about a close relative with an eating disorder, was advised against taking on someone whose history hinted that there might be similar elements.

The personal belief systems of students may become clear at some stage, and it may be a delicate matter to judge whether a devout believer will be able to work with a patient whose own beliefs or behaviours are challenging to the particular ideals of the student. I was surprised on at least one occasion that differences of conviction did not seem to interfere to any extent.

Students during their clinical years have to absorb a great deal of information and observe many differing specialisms and approaches to clinical work, and as so many new techniques have to be learned, it sometimes seems as if human contact with patients takes a back seat. The psychotherapy department is one place where things are different, but this means that some of what the students are learning and some of their assumptions about their future profession can and will be questioned. The three main areas of difference I find important are, first, to do with how one interviews the patient, in traditional medical terms, taking the history; second, the expectation that the doctor will carry the authority in the clinical situation; and last, the pressure on the doctor to be effective, to 'do something'.

Van Duuren has written of the difference for students between the 'medical' style of interviewing and relating to patients and the approach that we hope they will learn. They have already put in a lot of work in order to master the skill of medical history taking and to be able to do it quickly and efficiently, and they often want to practise it, so the idea of patiently waiting for the history to emerge, perhaps over weeks, is new and strange to them. The skill of listening to a patient, of being aware that the way that the story emerges may be as important as the story itself, develops slowly, and should the student for any reason become over-anxious, they may, like the keen and well-meaning student in Van Duuren's section, resort to an interrogatory style and inhibit the patient. A saying attributed to Michael Balint that I found useful and I often quote is

'If you ask questions, all you get is answers'. Most students understand this as meaning that useful information about another human being can be gathered just as much by observing their style of being and of relating as well as hearing their words, and indeed that the words they hear from the patients may be at odds with what they can observe, giving a clue to the patient's confusion or conflict. The facts of the history may be correct, and gathered in a short time; the effects of the history can frequently be observed through a much longer-term awareness of the patient's style of relating to the interviewer. However, even quite new habits can die hard, and the students have learned that finding out the hard facts about a patient quickly and accurately is what gains approval in the rest of their studies, so reverting to that style is tempting for them.

As Van Duuren has pointed out, medical students tend to be more open minded than young doctors and for that reason more able to think about different ways of relating to patients.

> One young man spelled it out to me very clearly by saying 'Something happens to people after they qualify. In a few weeks they become hardened and I find that people I was friends with aren't so nice any more. I'm scared that might happen to me'.

What he was observing was the effect on some young people of the exposure to the frightening responsibility that is the lot of the newly qualified doctor, and the development of defensive measures – the 'hardening off' – that many use to deal with the experience of painful helplessness in the face of desperate clinical situations which may compromise their sensitivity and even lead to a certain cynicism and emotional detachment that can be idealised as so-called 'clinical neutrality'. Students have yet to feel the weight of that responsibility and do not expect to 'know what to do', so can allow themselves to be curious and uncertain, and more able to learn.

The achievement of true clinical neutrality that is a non-intrusive and non-judgemental interest in the patient's situation, within a framework of basic goodwill towards the patient, is one of the aims of our scheme. I found that quite a lot of time was taken up with discussing it, both in relation to psychotherapy and also to medical practice in general. The usual expectation of a medical consultation is that the doctor will be the wise authority figure, giving advice, and the patient is the passive, obedient and even grateful recipient of that advice. Many students, faced with taking on a patient for themselves, are exceedingly concerned about their own inexperience and fear that to put themselves in the clinician's role as they understand it is falsely assuming a position they don't actually yet have. They do not feel wise, and are painfully aware of their ignorance.

When discussing the initial interview, for instance, I frequently found a wish in the student to introduce themselves to the patient with some humility, much as they might approach a patient when clerking them on a ward, 'Excuse me,

I'm only a medical student, would you mind if I talk to you?' being the kind of approach they are used to. In the face of this wish, as supervisor I found it an appropriate moment to introduce the concept of transference as an inevitable unconscious component of the relationship. I explain that although psychotherapy requires honesty and does not advocate lying to patients, who in any case have chosen to see a medical student, we are much more interested in studying the ways in which a therapist is seen and experienced by the patient, since that tells us more about the patient's way of relating. I explain that we try to withhold details about ourselves that might interfere too much with the emergence of the clinical picture we are interested in, and that might affect the pattern of transferences that the patient brings. The student can, without pretence of wisdom, focus on the patient and be interested in learning about him or her.

The students are thus frequently concerned about the possibility of being asked questions by patients, and whether they should answer them, or how to avoid them tactfully, while maintaining an atmosphere that might be described as basic friendliness without mutual confidences. They soon pick up that there is a difference between the intimacy of a friendship, in which confidences are exchanged, indeed vital to maintain the friendship, and the clinical situation in psychotherapy, in which a different kind of one-way intimacy can happen. Sometimes they find this a problem in practice, and are tempted to disclose something of their own, or to answer direct questions about themselves from the patient, particularly when they sense that the patient is vulnerable to a rebuff or a rejection. There can be a feeling that inviting confidences without offering them in return is somehow unfair, and to deal with the suspicion that they are engaging in something unfair, they may defend themselves by changing the general advice of the supervisor that they restrain themselves from personal disclosures to a strict rule, i.e. that patients must never under any circumstances learn anything at all about them. Taken to extremes, this can distort the students' experience.

> One girl stayed in the department at least half an hour after the patient had left for fear of catching the same bus home and being seen by the patient. Since the session did not finish until late she was very delayed and found herself going without supper in order to have time to study. As well as my own comments, discussion with her peer group was helpful, and eventually she was able to catch the right bus, only once seeing the patient outside the session. A nod of recognition was exchanged, and at the next session the patient expressed gratitude that she now knew that her therapist had a home to go to! The group proposed that the patient had picked up the therapist's anxiety and was relieved that it was reduced.

The common aim of all the students I came across was to become good doctors. To this end, they were already keen observers of the style of their teachers in clinical medicine and surgery. Most seemed ambitious to emulate those they considered not only good diagnosticians and practitioners, but also those who communicated sensitively, and whose concern for the patients they admired. Some also saw the more 'distant' style of some hospital doctors as being more professional, and were alarmed at the prospect of any emotion from either patient or clinician entering into the professional relationship. The topics of transference and countertransference can be explained in relation to these differences, and most students can begin to see them as inevitable aspects of clinical practice wherever it happens. They might even see that the 'distant' style is in fact a manifestation of countertransference in that it is a response to the fear of developing or recognising feelings that cannot be coped with about patients and the work. In this way a fear that the patient might burst into tears, accompanied by the conviction that should that happen the student would have somehow failed, could be transformed into a much more human reaction of empathy and the recognition that perhaps the sad patient has something real to cry about, and with this a more ordinary discussion in supervision about the pros and cons of offering him or her a tissue.

Concern about the emergence of negative feelings about patients is fairly easy to elicit – what if the patient turned out to be really unpleasant, hostile, complaining or even smelly? What if the patient was silent? How could the student maintain a neutral attitude if they found the patient unbearable? Dealing with these anticipatory anxieties is much helped by the scheme's pattern in which the new group of students join the group who are within sight of ending their year of psychotherapeutic work. The supervisor's advice that the inevitability of an emotional response to a patient – any patient – and the accompanying inevitability of the patient having both thoughts and feelings about the therapist may be a useful way of informing them theoretically about countertransference and transference. However, the confirmation with live examples from their colleagues reassures them that it is usual, acceptable, and can be worked with. In the face of their fears, the groups tend to find their own answers, and point out to each other that in the rest of their clinical studies, however unlikeable some of the patients might be, they find ways of relating to them and wanting to help them.

What is much more difficult to think about is the possibility of becoming fond of a patient, or worse still, being attracted to them.

One young man asked outright not to be given a young female patient, particularly if she turned out to be attractive, since he was anxious lest he fall in love with her. In fact, he fell foul of his own ambitions in another way; the passive, overweight and depressed male patient he did take on confided in him about a creative project he was secretly and privately engaged in. The student, almost unable to bear the grinding obstinacy and inactivity of his patient, became enthusiastic, and for a while hoped that he might have an undiscovered genius on his hands. It was only when the patient brought in some of his work on the project and the student recognised the banality of his efforts that he was able to admit the unrealistic nature of his own hopes for the patient and for himself. 'Some ugly ducklings are only ever going to be ugly ducks!' In the group he was able to recognise his disappointment and even laugh a little at himself, while beginning to value the fact that he was probably the only person who had ever shown much interest in the patient's inner life, and that in doing that he had given a positive experience to a man who was not just stubborn but also sad about his empty life.

In terms of the life of a teaching hospital the students come to learn that they are very much bottom of the medical hierarchy. Finding oneself being the principal clinician in a patient's treatment is a surprising and new experience, as is the idea that a patient will have thoughts and feelings about the therapist. Supervisors take very seriously the question of boundaries, and will emphasise early on the restraint and self-discipline necessary in a psychotherapeutic encounter. Students are used to being taught about self-discipline, so this is merely another version of what they are used to, albeit a different one. Being seen as an authority or even a parental figure is new to them, and they do not have the experienced psychotherapist's expectation that transferences are inevitable, or that the way they develop and manifest themselves can show not only something of the patient's inner world but also contains evidence of the patient's psychological developmental history. The extent to which students can pick these factors up varies; likewise, the awareness that unconscious factors operate in everyday life is something that some students naturally seem able to 'cotton on to', while some struggle, and others are bewildered and even uninterested.

Another pressure that many students feel derives from the assumption that it is a clinician's job to 'do something', and the ones who had the most difficulty in settling into the task were those whose keenness to be effective was the most urgent. They also want to know how psychotherapy works, and there can be a great deal of pressure to give advice, particularly when the student can see an easy solution to a difficult situation for the patient. Withholding advice seems cruel, and it may be necessary for the supervisor to explain that the patient's problem could be an inability to act on advice and our job is to find out why. Van Duuren asks 'What is therapy in this context?' and writes about the importance for the patient of being heard, and listened to, something that may never have happened to them before in quite that way. I have emphasised to the students that the patient also hears their own words, and by being in the presence of an attentive non-judgemental listener may allow the patient to make a temporary identification with that therapist/listener, so hearing their own story in a new way, allowing new thoughts and even alterations in feelings about themselves to happen. Knowing that the listener understands the patient's psychological pain can also relieve the loneliness that many patients feel.

The most dramatic change that I observed over a year of student psychotherapy was one in which a very quiet and rather motherly student listened
intently week after week to a middle-aged woman with a painful skin
condition who wept profusely as she told of her serial losses, of possessions,
country and relationship, and whose children rarely visited her. Each week
as I left the department following the students' seminar I saw this woman
whose skin was weeping even when her eyes were not as she waited for
her appointment. Although few interventions that might be called interpretations were made, the young woman who saw her so patiently and
recognised her pain, listened consistently and reported clearly each week,
including her own feelings of sympathy for and admiration of the patient
who, despite her grief, had survived so much. Towards the end of the year
I realised that the person sitting in the waiting room was unrecognisable.
Smiling, with a clear skin, she fitted the picture which was beginning to
emerge in the student's recent reports, of someone who was beginning to
make friends, had found a flat she liked, was beginning a new job, and
whose children seemed more willing to visit. Of course, at the end of the
year, the work included the consideration of the ending of the therapy, yet
another loss, but there were signs that she had managed to secure enough
positive elements in her life to sustain her through it.

The purpose of the Student Psychotherapy Scheme has always been to
facilitate the development of good communication and good doctor–patient
relationships, no matter what branch of medicine the student chooses to enter,
and for this reason teaching psychoanalytic theory is not its principal focus.
Where concepts derived from psychodynamic work apply, supervisors will take
the opportunity to explain their thinking, and students are usually interested:
this was the case with Van Duuren's student who asked about the Oedipus
complex, especially when the concept has immediate clinical impact, as
occurred on that occasion. My own hope was that the students might gain
familiarity with some thinking about the links between psychological health
and general health, the importance for psychological and indeed physical health
of early development, especially the development of relationships, an awareness
of transference and countertransference, with the concept of the tendency or
even compulsion to repeat, plus the awareness of defence mechanisms against
psychic pain of various sorts. By the end of the year, the students had faced
much about their patients and also about themselves, and the ending of the
relationship gave an opportunity of becoming aware of matters to do with loss
and mourning which were fairly easily understood, even when what had been
lost might have been a hope, an aspiration or a dream. Most of all, I hoped that
the students might come to understand the importance of the relationship
between clinician and patient no matter in what setting.

Nowadays, with recognition of the need for good doctor–patient communication, many medical schools address the same aim by providing practice

interviews for students, often with actors playing the role of patient. A variety of clinical situations can be played out and later discussed with their teachers, usually on a one-off basis. I learned that while the students on the whole enjoyed these sessions, they were well aware that these were not actual sufferers, and that they were not yet having to deal with real fear, bewilderment or pain, and that in these situations they carried no actual responsibility. The Student Psychotherapy Scheme, in contrast, gives an opportunity for continuing contact with a patient who has real difficulty of one sort or another, and who has hopes that this relationship will be helpful. The responsibility is real, and the patient they face has real problems. Their peers too, are in the same situation.

This is very different from listening to an actor, however skilled, and many of the doctors who have undertaken the scheme as students regard it as one of the most valuable experiences of their medical school training. Certainly for me, the teaching and the discussions that I had with the medical students taught me a great deal, and led me to respect the new generation and wish them well.

Chapter 3

Students' experiences of the UCL Student Psychotherapy Scheme

Jessica Yakeley, Robbie Bunt, Elsa Gubert and Caroline Hulsker

THE STUDENTS' EXPERIENCE

Jessica Yakeley

I know first hand what a powerful and enduring experience partaking in the Student Psychotherapy Scheme may be, having completed the scheme myself in the late 1980s. Taking on a real patient for psychotherapy with no prior experience seemed like a huge responsibility, and became one of my most significant and formative learning experiences at medical school. My patient was a woman presenting with difficulties in her marriage who was a decade older than me. I remember her seeming sophisticated, glamorous and worldly, and feeling quite intimidated. I wondered how on earth I could help her. I also remember feeling guilty that she had not been told that I was not a qualified therapist, which was the practice at that time. This, of course, has changed in that we are now more explicit and must gain the patient's informed consent that they are willing to be seen by a medical student. However, despite my anxieties, my patient quickly formed a trusting and dependent attachment to me, and I was powerfully introduced to the concepts of transference and acting out when she regressed and took a minor overdose when I could not see her for four weeks during an away attachment.

In this chapter, three doctors – Robbie Bunt, Elsa Gubert and Caroline Hulsker – all of whom also participated as medical students in the Student Psychotherapy Scheme, give a personal account of their recollections of the scheme and the influence it has had on their subsequent work as medical practitioners. Published accounts of medical students' personal experience of participating in the UCL Student Psychotherapy Scheme have existed in the literature from as early as 1981: several have been published in the British Medical Journal (Garner, 1981; Hoy, 2002; West, 2002) and others have been published elsewhere (Garner, 1985; Hampson, 1985; Prince, 1985; Hulsker, 2004; Antonelou, 2010). Although each of these accounts inevitably differs in reflecting the individual experiences and personalities of the students and patients concerned, they also illuminate and explore common themes and valued experiences that are echoed in the essays that follow. One of the skills learned through the scheme that is highlighted in many of these accounts is the development of a special kind of listening in the student. This involves the student having to shift from a more interrogative style of interviewing towards tolerating silences and being ready for what might emerge more spontaneously. This includes the student becoming more aware of their own particular style of relating to others and learning to be more aware of their anxieties and defensive strategies of interacting with patients:

> Patients can often be emotionally demanding, and this training has helped me learn how to deal with this.
>
> (Hoy, 2002, p. 57)

> The temptation to relieve the patient's tension and distress by reassurance diminished with time, and lengthy silences which appeared interminable at first became easier for both patient and therapist to tolerate.
>
> (Hampson, 1985, p. 95)

> Listening to someone and paying attention to what they want to say instead of thinking about my reply was not a simple task for me. I feared that I needed to come up with intelligent comments so that my patient did not think I was inadequate. When I realised that those sessions were not for me but for my patient, I immensely appreciated the importance of an extremely useful skill. I was made aware of the fact that the only way to help someone is to allow them to express their concerns and perspectives and adjust my approach according to their needs. On the ward, I found myself spending time truly listening to the patients instead of thinking of the list of symptoms I needed to go over. A better rapport was established and consultations became more efficient in terms of eliciting a relevant medical history.
>
> (Antonelou, 2010, p. 31)

> I now realise that during the settling-in period I tended to gather facts and attempted to rationalise problems into logical arguments. This form of intellectualising can be detrimental to therapy, sometimes evolving into a sort of word-game played at a higher level with total disregard for the wealth of material that the patient presents simply by being there. Euphemisms, silences, gestures and dreams gradually become more understandable and transferences may become more apparent. Recognising the patient's and one's own feelings gives access to a therapeutic barometer, perhaps reflecting how the patient interacts with other people.
>
> (Clifford, 1986, p. 368)

Such listening can evolve into a more sophisticated awareness of emotional states in both the student and the patient, and discovery that the student's feelings can be used as a tool to discern those of the patient. This is, of course, learning about the countertranference, a concept which these students found was useful in their interactions with patients in general:

> The way the therapist feels guides him to the way the patient feels.
>
> (Prince, 1985, p. 99)

> For those patients with physical illness, therapy improves the student's capability to care for them: he is able to listen, and can pick up the patient's feelings and use them to allay anxiety; he is sensitive to the subconscious in the patient and in himself, and, finally, he realises that the patient as a whole is his responsibility.
>
> (Garner, 1981, p. 798)

> If the patient's and one's own feelings are recognised, deeper anxieties may be anticipated, acknowledged and perhaps dealt with. This can only be achieved through constructive use of dialogue and not just by reassurance.
>
> (Clifford, 1986, p. 368)

Learning to differentiate one's own anxieties from those of the patient, and the critical role of the supervision meetings in facilitating this, are also highlighted by these students as important learning experiences:

> After several sessions, I was left very confused about the feelings I was experiencing during sessions. I believe that supervision played a very important role in helping me to clarify the origin of my feelings and use them as a source of insight into my patient's conflicts and defences.
>
> (Antonelou, 2010, p. 27)

Clifford (1986) recounts finding it difficult to concentrate in sessions with his patient and forgetting to bring his notes to supervision. Discussion in the supervision group allowed him to realise that his withdrawal from his patient was linked to recent material she had brought to her sessions regarding her uncle who had just died from emphysema. Clifford's own grandfather had recently become critically ill with the same condition, and had even been prescribed identical medication to his patient's uncle. His lack of focus and change of behaviour with his patient in the sessions defended him from awareness of his own anxiety about his relative.

Discovery of the transference and its potency may also be illuminating when the student realises what an important role they may rapidly assume in the patient's life. With this new knowledge students can begin to appreciate the significance of the level of trust and position of authority that a doctor can be endowed with by his or her patients, and the responsibility that caring for patients entails:

The way [my patient] reacts to me is focused on 'trying to please me in order to make me like her'. The possibility of me rejecting her causes a great deal of anxiety. This way of relating to me is similar to the way she reacts to her father and boss. Such an honest confession came as a shock to me. I felt intimidated and overwhelmed with the authority [my patient] was empowering me. I think those feelings were stemming from my insecurities of potentially being in the position to harm [my patient] by doing or saying something wrong.

(Antonelou, 2010, p. 26)

The scheme also teaches students to tolerate their own limitations and to modify their expectations regarding patient progress and notions of 'cure':

Being with my patient over an 18-month period was not always easy, or gratifying. I made mistakes. Progress was sometimes slow. This is, I believe, a fairly realistic approximation of the work of many clinicians. It is incredibly maturing. I realised that I did not have to be the perfect doctor. It is acceptable to have limitations, indeed important to be aware of them. My perspective on medicine has also changed. I no longer feel compelled to search for quick-fix remedies for physical ills. I have learned to approach patients holistically, and to appreciate the power of communication in healing.

(Hoy, 2002, p. 57)

The legacy of the scheme

Although I was already interested in pursuing psychiatry as a career, the experience of doing the Student Psychotherapy Scheme confirmed this as a career choice, and was also influential in my later decision to train as a psychoanalyst. However, although many of the students who participate in the scheme do end up as psychiatrists, its primary aim is to teach students about the doctor–patient relationship with an emphasis on attaining a deeper understanding of the role of emotions. This is useful for all future doctors, whatever their clinical specialty. When we looked at the career choices of medical students who had participated in the Student Psychotherapy Scheme we found that many students had gone into general practice, hospital medicine and surgery (see Chapter 8). They reported how the scheme stood out for them as one of the most worthwhile experiences of medical school, and how much it had helped them in communicating with their patients to this day. Many also wished to be remembered to their supervisors. None of the three contributors to this chapter became psychiatrists after doing the scheme: Bunt and Gubert became GPs, and Hulsker is a paediatric surgeon. However, they all describe how the experience of seeing a patient for supervised psychotherapy as a medical student influenced their relationships with patients years later in positive and sometimes unexpected ways.

The scheme may also forge a special kinship between those who have been involved, illustrated in Robbie Bunt's account below of forming a GP practice with another ex-student of the scheme, and also in an experience that I had recently. I was appointed as Director of Medical Education for my trust a few years ago, and was feeling somewhat anxious about my first Deanery inspection visit. The board room seemed full of important people from my own trust and the Deanery, all looking very serious. One of the deans looked vaguely familiar, and she recognised me as well. We eventually worked out that she had been a medical student in the same medical school, and then that she had also done the Student Psychotherapy Scheme and had been in the same supervision group as me. We started talking about the scheme, how it had helped her in her work as an endocrinologist, and then the woman chairing the meeting, a genito-urinary physician, revealed that she had also done the scheme a few years earlier. At this point, the medical director said that he had also done it, and the only people left in the room who had not, were the chief executive and the finance director!

ON BEING HELD

Robbie Bunt

In the 1980s I saw a psychotherapy patient once weekly for 1 year as part of the UCL Student Psychotherapy Scheme. Whilst a lot of the detail of the work is forgotten, what I remember clearly is the last session in which my patient, a young woman whose problems stemmed from an emotionally abusive relationship with her father, brought a dream about hands holding her as she fell asleep. In the supervision group that followed, my supervisor interpreted this as a sign of how my patient had been 'held' in the therapy. I would like to use this as a theme for how my time as a student in medical school was held by my experience of the scheme, and how the early experience of holding a patient in a therapeutic relationship has influenced my work now as a GP.

For the last 20 years I have been a partner in a busy inner-city general practice. One of my three partners in the practice is also an ex-student of the scheme and we went through medical school together. We pride ourselves as a practice on trying to provide a 'usual doctor system', with continuity of care for our patients wherever possible. As a medical student I did an intercalated BSc in psychology in my third year, and following this I joined the Student Psychotherapy Scheme during my clinical years. I left medical school unsure if I wanted a career in general practice or psychiatry, so started my journey on a vocational GP training scheme. I went on from this to a general psychiatry rotation but after about a year had realised that the sort of psychiatry I really enjoyed was what was found in general practice. I became a partner in the practice where I now work in the early 1990s. I have been fortunate enough to complete a Diploma in Psychoanalytical Psychotherapy at the Tavistock

Clinic in the late 1990s and to be part of a Balint group at the Tavistock during this time. We are a training practice for GPs and also teach medical students on their primary care attachment. I have become more and more involved in medical politics, and try to use my influence from this work to protect what I see as the core values of general practice in a system that seems to ignore and value only counting what can be counted.

I would like to first go back to being at medical school and think about my experience of the scheme in relation to this. I am sure I am not the only doctor to remember medical school, especially the clinical years, as a quite brutal experience. The rapid transfer from one clinical firm to another did not allow any relationship to develop between student and teacher, and indeed teaching seemed often an annoyance to those who were teaching. I can recall a Saturday morning ward round when I had been up all night in the Accident and Emergency Department the previous night, being asked in front of an embarrassed patient if I had 'ever opened a medical textbook in my life.' This was before the days of having individual tutors, and of course the Student Psychotherapy Scheme filled a void and provided the ongoing support and relationship I needed. For once there was a consultant who seemed genuinely interested in me as a person, in my thoughts and ideas, someone whom I met up with once a week over a prolonged period of time and therefore with whom I developed a relationship. The supervision group allowed me for the first time to have a safe place to discuss my worries and concerns, both with the supervisor and my peers. I believe this sowed the seed of that important ability to be able to discuss cases with colleagues in an open and non-judgemental way.

More importantly, I think the group, and my relationship with it, held me through the somewhat cold and barren landscape of the clinical years of medical school. My mother developed breast cancer during this period of my studies. I am sure that my supervisor was the only member of the medical school staff who was aware of this and I much valued his support and kind words during this time. Such life events that can happen to us all, and that are so important to process, are much easier when there is another who under-stands what one is going through. So while my patient felt held by the therapy, I believe I was held by the scheme as I progressed through medical school.

How does the Student Psychotherapy Scheme relate to my work now as a GP? I have always viewed some of what I do in general practice as a kind of protracted psychotherapy that lasts for many years. While in inner-city practice we see our practice population turn over by approximately 30% each year, there is a steady cohort of patients and families who have remained with me as their GP for nearly 20 years now. The patient and their family are, when this works well, held by the GP and indeed by the institution of the practice itself. Fundamental to this is a 'usual doctor system' – we try to encourage continuity of care by giving each patient a named usual doctor who will hopefully be the doctor they most often consult with, barring holidays, who deals with all their repeat prescriptions and any incoming letters or results. This gives our practice a familiar face and allows for the opportunity for relationships to develop over time. In survey results we generally do well in such measures as 'ability to see the doctor you want to see' or 'feeling listened to'. Maybe we do not do so well on other measures, for example 'the ability to get an appointment within 24 hours', and indeed this is the constant challenge of modern general practice: the patient's agenda is often at odds with what the government expects and therefore rewards us for doing, and the practice that does not take heed of this will unfortunately not survive financially. There is little reward currently in our contract for encouraging continuity of care, yet I believe it is only with this that relationships between doctors and patients can develop, so that patients can feel held and that other agendas can be allowed to emerge.

What did I learn from the scheme that relates to my work as a GP? I think first and foremost it is the skill of listening. Being able to sit in a room with another person and hear their thoughts, with empathy but without the need to rush into saying something or doing something, like writing a prescription for instance or making a referral, is a valuable skill.

Over many years in a practice, relationships and trust develop between patient and general practitioner, and transference and countertransference phenomena occur. Sometimes I think these can be safely and usefully commented on in the general practice setting, and I will in those situations sometimes make an interpretation which can take the consultation to another level. I do not tell my patients what to call me, but try to reflect to myself what it means when I am called 'doc', or by my first name after only maybe one or two consultations, or by a much more formal use of my title and surname.

I try to think about the setting and remember back to the days of the scheme, rearranging my student room at UCH every week back to how it should look for my patient. Now I have my own room, and apart from interruptions of daily GP life which disturb the consultation, this is not so much an issue. However, I do try to keep something of the texture of the setting – somewhat bland and devoid of any personal artifacts, so that as far as possible there are few preconceptions of who I am or might be. I sometimes wonder how it must feel, for example, to an infertile couple coming into a consulting room to be bombarded with pictures of the doctor's children on family holidays.

The issue of boundaries is of particular importance in general practice, and I believe my training in this difficult area began with what I learned from the scheme about the boundaries of the psychotherapeutic relationship. I have often seen other doctors get drawn into behaviours which I feel sure are helpful neither to them nor to their patients, yet it is easy to get drawn into inappropriate actions unless one is aware of and keeps an eye open for boundary issues. Similarly, requests from one's own friends or family members to be drawn into being their GP are often difficult and sometimes met with annoyance when the request is politely refused and it is suggested that they should see their own GP. Being able to have difficult conversations and respecting personal and professional boundaries in this are a fundamental part of the landscape of good general practice.

There is much I am sure I have forgotten about my experience all those years ago, and much that was learned or that sustained me in my training that I have taken for granted. Aside from the friendship of my fellow students and the ongoing relationships from those days which enrich my life, the Student Psychotherapy Scheme is the part of my studies that I hold most dear in recollection of medical school days. In conclusion, I hope I have been able to demonstrate how being held in a therapeutic relationship as my patient was acts as a metaphor for the medical student being held by the scheme, and also the 'holding' of patients that occurs in general practice.

A BREATH OF LIFE IN A TIME OF SPIRITUAL HUNGER

Elsa Gubert

The Student Psychotherapy Scheme at UCL offers an unparalleled opportunity to accompany a patient along their difficult journey. The student learns first hand how much power there can be in active listening and how slow the process of change can be.

For me, as a 23-year-old medical student, the scheme conveyed a powerful message. It told me that my interaction with patients was important, not just for my own learning, but as part of the patient's journey. The Psychotherapy Department clearly believed that my colleagues and I had within us a far-reaching tool, which we could harness whatever our chosen career was to be. Above all I felt that despite being one of over 300 students, what I thought mattered. For a few sacred hours every week, I could put away my textbooks and really listen to my patient. In supervision, I could talk about my own personal experience of seeing her and my thoughts and interpretations would be listened to with great interest.

The scheme gave us time to think. It gave us time to sit back and really look at our patients and see what might have led them to be who they are, and how this might impact on their health and their relationships. Our realisations owed much to the quality of listening we experienced from our supervisors. I suspect that many of the students on the scheme had never been listened to like this before, and I am sure we all became better listeners as a result.

When I met my patient 'Emily' I had been attending a supervision group for 8 weeks. However, I remained apprehensive. How would a 23-year-old student help a 50-year-old woman with a longstanding history of depression, entrenched in abusive relationships and struggling with symptoms of chronic fatigue syndrome? Emily was reaching out for help having recently lost her father and separated from her long-term partner. My supervisor warned me that I might see little change over the course of the year, and I knew this would be challenging for me. I wondered whether I would be able to do more than support Emily through this difficult phase of her life.

From the outset, I was amazed to see how readily Emily accepted me as her therapist. She never commented about my age or lack of experience, and we very quickly established a warm relationship. Emily turned out to be a highly insightful person. Throughout the therapy she spontaneously made links between mind and body, feelings and actions. She also attended very regularly and was rarely late.

At the start of therapy, Emily was entwined in a complex web of relationships, which often led her to feel weak and victimised. She spent a lot of time looking after others, and rarely expressed her own needs. As the therapy progressed, she took a little more distance from her family, which allowed her to spend more time working on healthy friendships rather than being sucked into painful conflicts within her family.

Initially, Emily's symptoms of chronic fatigue syndrome seemed to get worse. She felt physically drained and started to complain of nausea. However, as time went on these symptoms began to fade. Emily made useful links between her fatigue and her contact with her family. Whenever Emily saw her youngest daughter she felt exhausted and nervous. She realised that as a child she had been conditioned to suppress her emotions. She saw that situations which stifled her feelings often led to a worsening of her physical symptoms.

Half way through the therapy there was a violent break in the relationship between Emily and her youngest daughter. This plunged Emily into a very dark mood. She began to have thoughts of self harm and mentioned fleeting suicidal thoughts. I was worried that I might not be able to contain the crisis. I spoke to my supervisor, and with Emily's consent we contacted her GP. Fortunately, Emily soon felt better when limited contact with her daughter was re-established. This was my first experience of 'safety netting' and writing to a doctor in a professional capacity. I experienced a new sense of agency and of responsibility to patients. Interestingly, the very events that were so painful for Emily were pivotal in allowing her and her daughter to move forward and loosen their excessively close ties.

For me, Emily was a very intelligent, insightful lady. Although she sometimes asked whether I could 'cope' with seeing her again the following week, my time with her was very valuable to me. Perhaps her continued contact with someone who appreciated her and listened to her helped Emily remember what it is to feel valued.

As the ending of the therapy approached, Emily spoke of the future with a sense of optimism. I felt more cautious, knowing that Emily would continue to struggle with the upheavals that are inevitable in a large family full of troubled characters. I was sad to hear my supervisor tell me she had taken a turn for the worse soon after our relationship ended. This may have been a reaction to separation and ending the therapy, a time when commonly patients may experience a temporary resurgence of their symptoms and difficulties that they originally presented with.

I left the scheme with a more realistic perspective on healing. I realised that psychological change takes time, and we cannot rush it, whether with counselling or medications. I became more comfortable dealing with silence, with tears and with very sensitive discussions, for instance around sexual relationships. I also realised just how much insight patients can have, and this has encouraged me to listen to their own interpretations before voicing my own.

During the long dry years of hospital medicine there was very little room for this precious form of listening and few continued relationships with patients. Few were the clinicians who accepted and encouraged us to express our emotions and allow our personality into our work. Perhaps this is necessary in the fast-paced, stressful environment of hospital medicine. The scheme showed me the way back to a career that attributed much more importance to the emotions of both doctor and patient. I knew I had to choose a profession that valued the doctor–patient relationship more than it did the prescription pad.

My psychotherapy scheme supervisor introduced me to the work of Michael Balint. In fact the UCL Psychotherapy Department helped me towards the funding of a place at the Balint Oxford weekend in 2004, where I met many like-minded general practitioners. Without a doubt, participating in the Student Psychotherapy Scheme clarified my professional aspirations. It is not a coincidence that I went on to apply to the Whittington vocational training scheme, which has a strong emphasis on Balint work as well as a particularly holistic approach to the person and work of the general practitioner. I felt that here in the Psychotherapy Department I was learning meaningful principles about humanity that would inform my perception of patients throughout my career.

Looking back at my experience of the psychotherapy scheme, I realise that my relationship with Emily still stands out as truly unique in my career so far. Even now as a fully qualified GP, I work in the context of fragmented 10-minute appointments. I have as yet never worked in one place for more than 18 months, and what I experienced with Emily seems like a dream. I can hardly remember what it felt like to have the luxury of 50 minutes with a patient undisturbed every week.

The experience of this luxury has made me much more curious about my patients. It has helped me to build the space in my short consultations to hear something about their inner worlds. I believe I am a better doctor for it, even if I do often run late! I chose a career in medicine because I wanted to understand health and illness and help steer patients towards health. The scheme showed me what I might strive for in my career as a general practitioner: meaningful relationships with patients that allow both doctor and patient to grow.

FROM STUDENT PSYCHOTHERAPIST TO PAEDIATRIC SURGEON

Caroline Hulsker

When I came to London for my clinical medical studies, I obviously had several expectations and fears. My expectations were high: I was to finally come into contact with patients, be exposed to multiple clinical problems and a variety of hospitals around central London. I was excited to have successfully completed my undergraduate studies and be able to put my knowledge into practice. The prospect of meeting patients and being on the hospital wards filled me with excitement.

However, I also feared that throughout medical training, time with patients would be relatively short and as communication would be of the essence, I was afraid that I would not be able to communicate well and establish a proper rapport with patients. I wondered how well a medical student could get to know a patient, and whether patient contact would be limited to single events or whether we could follow a patient throughout the course of their illness. I also wondered whether we were supposed to focus on the medical problem itself and whether it was appropriate to ask questions beyond the presenting illness at hand. Furthermore, I was well aware that a medical student does not have a position of responsibility within the medical team caring for a patient, and that this could well mean that a patient would not want to speak to a medical student. And what influence would I, as a student, have on the patient?

At the same time, I was fascinated by the concept of illness. What would it mean to patients to bear a chronic illness or to fall ill acutely? What mental baggage would patients be bringing to the hospital, and would it affect their illness, or their recovery? Would medical students be able or allowed to delve into these mental processes behind the patient's illness?

Coming from a family of general practitioners, dentists and a chest physician, I was used to medical issues being discussed throughout my childhood. My grandfather had been the only doctor in a small rural town. Hearing stories from him, I realised that knowing family relations and the history of patients and their children and grandchildren added much value to the way my grandfather was able to treat these entire families. He knew stories from patients who had not even told their wife what they told him. My grandfather saw the lives of his patients, their children and sometimes grandchildren unfold. What did this mean to him? Did this affect the way he treated each patient? Would I be able to establish a practice in the same way?

I went into my clinical medical studies having no idea what field of medicine I would eventually go into. I very much enjoyed absorbing everything and learning about the link between certain illnesses, especially when they overlapped in, for example, the medical and surgical realms. I was looking forward to the prospect of 3 years of clinical studies and being exposed to every field.

Coming across the possibility of participating in the Student Psychotherapy Scheme, I was delighted at the chance to see a patient on a regular basis and for this to not necessarily be a purely medical experience. I knew that the scheme would be a unique opportunity to have a position of responsibility. Knowing that a patient would come in every week to speak to you, and no one else, was something that did not happen anywhere else during medical training. Through weekly sessions with a patient, the patient would be able to feel different, maybe even better. The patient and I would be able to develop a relationship and this would enable the patient to reveal thoughts and feelings to an extent that I had never experienced in medical training.

I was reassured by the fact that the scheme had been running for years, as was explained to us. The set-up had been thought through carefully and had evolved over time. Getting to grips with some basic principles of psychoanalysis and psychotherapy gave me a foundation. Nevertheless, I was anxious at the prospect of meeting my patient for the first time. This was also well prepared for. Not only did we, as a group, consider how we would greet our patient and introduce ourselves, but we also discussed how we would tackle questions about who we were and what our exact position within the Psychotherapy Department was.

When the weekly sessions started, it was a process of quick learning and understanding. We started by discussing the condition of the patient allocated to me: she suffered from a chronic mild depression and had gone through a protracted grieving process. My having an open and relatively unprepared mind as the therapist in the early sessions contributed to the patient's feeling of freedom in speaking to me.

At first there was hesitation on my patient's behalf at having been assigned to a student. This was, it turned out, to do with the fact that she had issues with not feeling taken seriously throughout her life. Entering a Student Psychotherapy Scheme, rather than seeing a 'regular' psychotherapist, therefore, was a starting point which led to the patient opening up about this feeling. As well as this being a challenge and making me feel anxious about the expectations I thought I had to live up to, discussing the patient's concerns created trust between us when we spoke about it in the first few sessions.

Soon after this, I began to feel that seeing my patient regularly was allowing her to open up and actually speak extremely freely in my presence. She confessed that she would not open up to anyone, not even to her family or close friends, in the same way. This instilled a sense of responsibility in me I had not encountered in my medical training to date, and would not until I was much further advanced in my postgraduate specialist training.

Furthermore, it also made me realise that spending time with a patient in a one-on-one setting can have a great effect on the life of him or her. I started making an effort in my regular medical training to spend time, sometimes only for 5 to 15 minutes, to sit with patients on the ward and speak to them. The effect of this was noticeable straight away. To this day, I enjoy going to the ward and, if it is possible, to spend extra time with patients.

As the weekly sessions continued, more issues that my patient coped with unraveled. I was surprised to see how this happened with hardly any of my own input, or so it felt. The space and time the scheme offered facilitated this process, and again this was something I had not experienced in my regular medical training. I became surer of myself as a listener, and realised the power of listening and the power of silence. In the outpatient setting or on the wards, I now often let silence enter the conversation, without being afraid of an awkward moment. I am always surprised at what comes out of these moments, and continue to implement this in my daily practice.

Finally, admitting that some aspects of patients' problems are beyond the scope and comfort zone of the student is an integral part of the scheme. It became clear that my patient suffered from some longstanding problems she had never discussed with her GP or counsellor, and that these issues were not known to the Psychotherapy Department either, before her involvement in the scheme. When this became clear, and when I brought these issues up in the group discussion, it was extremely useful to be advised and to know I had full support of my supervisor and the department. Eventually it was decided that, for some particular issues, my patient should be referred to another department, and I received a lot of advice and guidance on how to best proceed to discuss this with my patient. I felt safe and within my comfort zone because of this.

The weekly group discussions in the supervision meetings added to my reassurance and allowed others to reflect and advise on the process with my patient, and vice versa. The input of the psychiatrist leading the group discussions was invaluable in this and I am extremely grateful for his advice and guidance throughout the scheme. It created a safe environment for the students, and thereby also for the patients.

Reflecting on my year in the Student Psychotherapy Scheme, I believe this gave me so much more than anything regular medical training could have offered. I am extremely grateful that I was allowed to take part in the scheme, and to share my thoughts about it afterwards.

After finishing medical training and foundation house officer years, I worked in Australia for a year, and then returned to my home country, the Netherlands, where I completed a surgical training programme. I feel I have become a surgeon who enjoys the ward and outpatient clinical settings just as much as the operating theatre. I appreciate being able to have long discussions with patients and their families about the prospects of their illness and their feelings about surgical treatment or the decision not to perform surgery. I feel the choice to go into paediatric surgery is partly based on the fact that, in this field, there is never just one patient and the doctor–patient setting always involves family members or guardians. It is essential to make patients and their families feel that they can speak freely and to allow them to show their emotions. Even as a surgeon, I can feel the strong influence of the Student Psychotherapy Scheme.

Chapter 4

The Bristol Student Psychotherapy Scheme

Ray Brown and Thanos Tsapas

BEGINNINGS

Ray Brown

The Student Psychotherapy Scheme, which began in Bristol in 1996, has been a transformative experience for students and teachers. I was appointed in 1993 to the United Bristol Healthcare Trust as a consultant medical psychotherapist to set up a tertiary psychodynamic psychotherapy service. I was the first consultant psychotherapist to be appointed to this trust. Initially, there was no team, no base, and no history or culture of psychoanalytic psychotherapy – it was a complete *tabula rasa*. However, a number of consultant psychiatrist colleagues were enthusiastic about developing psychotherapy and were key to the subsequent development of our scheme.

Two consultant psychotherapy colleagues based within adjoining trusts already knew about the Student Psychotherapy Scheme at University College London (UCL). One had been a student on the UCL scheme and the other had a detailed knowledge about it. My own experience was of being a supervisor for the UCL Student Psychotherapy Scheme for about 3 years during a placement at University College Hospital (UCH) that was part of my higher training in psychotherapy at the Portman Clinic. This experience inspired me to develop a similar scheme in Bristol. This new scheme was first based in Barrow Hospital, on the outskirts of Bristol. It was a hospital without any direct commercial bus service or any suitable rooms available for patients to be seen by students. I discussed these problems with my consultant colleagues, who had offices, as I did, in a separate wing with six rooms. They supported the idea for the scheme and agreed to vacate their offices and clear their desks of any confidential material just before 5pm each Monday. There was a seminar room at the end of the block that could seat a group of 10 to 12 people comfortably. My secretary also agreed to rearrange her time so that she could be present until 6.30pm. When these arrangements began to look workable, I decided that I would try to pilot the scheme, voluntarily devoting 3 hours on Monday nights between 5 and 8pm.

David Mumford, who was a senior lecturer in the Department of Mental Health at Bristol University, with responsibility for the psychiatry teaching programme for medical students, knew about the UCL scheme and was a key figure in developing the scheme in Bristol. His close involvement with educational developments within the medical school and his psychiatric background helped him to provide the necessary support for this project. To give the scheme an official status in the undergraduate curriculum, and to enable the students to receive educational credit for the time they spent, students had the option to submit a written report on their experience as a 'Special Study Module' (SSM) as promoted by the GMC to encourage educational breadth beyond the core medical curriculum.

We had discussions about where the scheme would best fit in the 5-year undergraduate medical programme. Although there was designated SSM time in Year 3, it was considered desirable that students should have had previous experience of psychiatry before embarking on the scheme and so the fourth year (i.e. their second clinical year) was preferred. The medical students were informed of the course in the early summer, with a starting date set in September. Their responses were usually all in before the medical students' summer holidays. Third-year students were not excluded, but most of the students were fourth year, having done their psychiatry attachment. This is in contrast to the UCL scheme which takes third-year students (first-year clinical students) who have not yet done their psychiatric placements.

Between 30 and 40 medical students attended our first meetings, which were held in a large conference room in Barrow Hospital. Transport to the hospital was by car, with those students having cars giving others a lift. This arrangement of providing lifts was remarkably coordinated, even from early on. These meetings, which I led, ran for an hour and a half and were not particularly structured, with topics for discussion determined by the medical students' wishes. As a theoretical starting point, I used the writings of David Malan, and the group would together read out loud chapters from his book, *Individual Psychotherapy and the Science of Psychodynamics* (Malan, 1999). Later, students had access to a wide range of reading material and a free discussion would follow. Medical students were encouraged to discuss anything interesting or upsetting that they had experienced so far in their training. One student told us about a patient being told bluntly, without any preparation, that he had a tumour and that he was not expected to live very long. Using this sort of experience we tried to explore concepts such as identification, transference, countertransference and empathy. Later I introduced role play into the group. Medical students, following a suitable briefing, would play the role of a therapist or patient. I also took part in this role play, which included the actions of going to an imaginary waiting room to greet a patient and leading them into the therapy room. The form of address, introduction and seating arrangements were discussed, as was the exchange between the imaginary patient and the imaginary psychotherapist. Role play was kept relatively brief, lasting no more than 10 minutes. This helped to reduce the anxiety about the possible forthcoming initial meetings with a real patient and also stimulated interest and discussion in the student group.

The medical students were told from the start that there would be only 12 places on the scheme, with some of the students included as observers but not actually treating patients. The responsibility and commitment involved in doing psychotherapy was discussed in various ways. Students had often complained to me in these discussions that they felt they had no role or responsibility during their training and that they often felt infantilised by their teachers. Some medical students, when the extent of responsibility and time commitment was clarified, felt unable to make that commitment; others, however, welcomed both the responsibility and the challenge. The initial contact with patients was in November and continued until the beginning of the medical students' summer holidays in July of the following year. A substantial number continued to attend, and viewed the seminars as an introduction to psychotherapy, but with the limited number of places available for students to see a patient, some students dropped out of the scheme.

During the last seminar those students who wished to continue made this clear, and sometimes as many as 20 remained. By this time I felt I had got to know the group and had heard them all talk and express their thoughts about clinical matters. Sometimes it was clear that certain of them had too strong an anti-authoritarian attitude or were too anxious and I was concerned that these problems might give rise to later difficulties in supervising them. Since there were invariably more medical students than places, the selection method we arrived at, which was thought to be fair in the circumstances, was to draw lots for places on the scheme.

The patients, who were either referred by my consultant psychiatrist colleagues or came from our group waiting list, were selected on the basis that they did not carry a risk of suicide, psychosis or aggressive behaviour. When I met any patient referred for an assessment by a consultant psychiatrist, I would inform them about the Student Psychotherapy Scheme, explaining that they might be seen if they wished on this scheme by a medical student after they had had two meetings with this student. If patients were already on the waiting list built up from tertiary referrals, I would meet them to outline the details of the scheme and explain that their decision about whether or not to proceed would not affect their chances of being considered for long-term individual or group therapy.

Once we had selected those students who were to go on to see patients or to become observers, we moved from the conference room to the wing where the seminar room and treatment rooms were located. In this new setting a number of further practical matters were addressed. There was a need to ensure the security and safety of the arrangements. I told the medical students that I would always be present in the building while they were seeing patients, and would be available if there was any concern. I informed them that there was also an on-call psychiatrist available if needed. I gave all the medical students my home telephone number and said they could call me at any time if they felt worried about their patient. The students all exchanged mobile telephone numbers, so that any student could quickly communicate with other students and myself to pass on a message if for any reason they were delayed or could not attend a session. Practical arrangements regarding the students' ease of transport to the hospital to ensure punctuality, and the suitability and layout of the rooms in which they would see their patients, were also discussed in detail prior to starting.

While these arrangements were being made, potential patients were discussed. I would bring case notes to the meeting and ask a medical student to present one of the cases. The students would then discuss the case and were encouraged to share their feelings as fully as possible. In this way it was possible to consider their countertransference responses to the patients. I found that the students would make connections to other people and experiences in their lives, and so be able to get an idea of whether or not they wished to work with a patient. Usually one of the group would clearly express a wish to work with a particular patient. Initially there was a tendency for some of the students to hold back from taking on a patient so they could see how their colleagues got on with their first case.

Once a case had been allocated, the students of their own accord divided into two equal groups. One group of four supervisees, with often a fifth person observing, would meet for supervision at 5pm, and see their patients at 6.10pm. The second supervision group saw their patients at 5pm and attended for supervision at 6pm. At 7pm, both supervision groups met together until 7.30pm to share any additional difficulty or issues they wished to discuss. This was an extremely compact arrangement for meetings, giving students who were seeing patients at 5pm only 10 minutes or so to write an outline of their notes for their subsequent presentation if they were due to present at 6pm. The medical students also only had about 30 minutes a fortnight to discuss their case. The medical students felt that they learned from and valued hearing colleagues discuss cases and some of the issues could be generalised to their own case.

The students saw their patients for 12 to 20 sessions, always informing the patient about the length of the therapy at its commencement. These arrangements became a regular pattern over the ensuing years, but managing this scheme alone proved to be a great responsibility.

Luckily, there were further developments. David Mumford became the Director of Medical Education for Bristol University Medical School in 1998. The medical students had been giving good feedback about their experience on the Psychotherapy Scheme and David's enlightened view was that students should be encouraged to follow their study interest in medicine, which would lead not only to educational benefits but development as a person and the development of capacity rather than just competence. Together with an increase in the medical school's intake of students, new national funding arrangements came into place with the development of Service Increment for Teaching (SIFT) funding for NHS staff involvement in teaching medical students for whom our scheme was renamed as a Student Selected Component (SSC), which now made it part of the medical curriculum. We now had money (from SIFT funding) to pay for one consultant medical psychotherapist session to run the scheme. In addition to these financial changes the student clinical placements became more consistently closer to our unit. So it became easier for students to come to the department to see their patients and not have to travel from so far away. Also, in 2000, the scheme was relocated in the Susan Britton Wills Unit, a community mental health centre in which the tertiary psychotherapy services for south Bristol were based. Here, there was a receptionist who worked till late on Monday evenings, a dedicated waiting room and a suite of therapy rooms. This site was also familiar to the patients, since I had initially assessed them there. Other senior staff became involved in providing supervision.

The development of the SSCs in the MB ChB programme was extremely beneficial: with the development of the scheme as an SSC there was a requirement for the students to write an essay, which helped them to consolidate their learning and to process their experience of seeing a patient. This was greatly valued by the medical students. I marked all their SSCs, but with hindsight, I would have liked to have had much more time with each medical student to discuss their work. My involvement in running the scheme ended in July 2009 with my retirement from the NHS.

DEVELOPMENTS

Thanos Tsapas

When I was appointed I was excited to be responsible for continuing the long tradition of the scheme and to have the opportunity to work with medical students in this way. Since then, the Psychotherapy Service has been incorporated within a Bristol-wide Psychological Therapies Service. These changes, however, have not affected the scheme, which has continued to run every year and which has remained very popular with the students. Participating in it has become a topic for discussion in medical student circles and the ones who have already completed it work hard to advertise it to other students. In response to an increased demand for places, it became possible in 2012–13 to expand the scheme so that it could accommodate up to 11 students instead of the original six. Some aspects of the scheme have remained exactly the same as in previous years and some have changed. One of the most significant and potent aspects of the scheme are the practical arrangements for supervision and seeing patients which have maximised its containing capacity. Students have commented on several occasions that the ready availability of the supervisor by email and mobile phone outside the normal regular supervision time has significantly helped them to deal with their patients' presenting difficulties and risk and with their own anxieties.

For example, one student interrupted a supervision group and reported that her patient had left half way through his session after a difficult discussion, where he had spoken about sexual abuse he had suffered in childhood. The patient then returned to the consulting room and revealed that he had taken an overdose, but insisted on leaving the session and the building. The therapist and I managed to have a discussion with the patient, which allowed him to reflect on what had happened in the session prior to the overdose. He then agreed to be transferred by ambulance to the nearest A&E department. The patient was able to attend the next session and continue with the therapy for another 2 months until the agreed ending date. Two months later I reviewed him and further arrangements were made for him to have individual psychotherapy for another 2 years. The following year the patient became suicidal and again contemplated taking an overdose at around the same time that he had been in this therapy. It transpired that this was a significant anniversary related to his past experiences of abuse.

Our scheme is now limited to fourth-year students, which means that they have all had an experience of a 9-week psychiatric placement in the previous year before joining it. This placement may stimulate the students' interest in the scheme and it has often been the case that this has been a deciding factor in expressing a keen interest in it and applying for it. It is difficult to know whether an unsatisfactory or even traumatic psychiatric placement may deter some other students from applying. An added benefit of accepting only the fourth- rather than the third-year students is that they have accumulated some clinical experience and so will have developed some skills that could be useful when seeing patients for psychotherapy. Because the students have had substantial training and practice in an illness-and-symptom-orientated approach to patients, they sometimes struggle to let go of a history taking (questioning) technique when they see their psychotherapy patients. However, by limiting the scheme to the fourth year, we deprive these students of being in a group in which there is a mixture of years: in a mixed-year group new students can share their initial anxieties with older members of the group, who are already familiar with these problems.

The other aspect of the scheme which has remained largely unchanged is the preparatory period that usually lasts for 10 weeks from late September to the beginning of December of each academic year. During this time the students begin to reflect in the group setting on important questions such as 'What is psychotherapy?', on their role in caring for patients, their identity as medical students, the difference between medical and psychotherapy settings, and the ethical issues arising in both settings. Particular emphasis is placed on professional boundaries and the 'setting', and ideas such as projective identification, transference and countertransference are introduced. These sessions contribute greatly to alleviating the students' initial anxieties about seeing their patients, increase their confidence and enhance their ability to learn from others and remain reflective. Such a preparatory period also allows the students to test their motivation and commitment to the scheme.

In 2012–13 we were able to expand the scheme when we received additional monies from SIFT funds generated by increased numbers of SSC students, which paid for an additional consultant medical psychotherapist session. However, this expansion of the scheme highlighted and intensified a pre-existing difficulty in finding enough suitable patients for the students. As a result of many service changes in General Adult Psychiatry and the Psychological Therapies Service, because of re-commissioning of the mental health services in Bristol, it has become increasingly difficult to find suitable patients for the students. We are now dealing with patients who present with multiple and complex needs, co-morbidity and high risk. This difficulty has been overcome in two ways: first, it was agreed that the Liaison Psychiatry Department of the local general hospital could refer directly to the Psychological Therapies Service to cover some of the students' and other trainees' needs; second, six of the students were placed at a local GP practice and began to see patients who had been referred directly from the general practitioners working there.

These new arrangements with the GP practice were the result of a number of discussions with two local GPs. I assessed and obtained consent to see a student from all the referred patients in this practice. They all agreed to be seen by a student and started their weekly sessions. Most of these patients said how much they valued the psychotherapy being provided within the same place, even in the same room, as they had been seen by their GP many times before. It seems that the accessibility, familiarity and the holding quality of this environment played a significant role in allowing them to engage in therapy. Some of the patients added that they would not have contemplated seeing a therapist outside the practice. Despite the fact that the assessment process in this new setting, and the liaising with the referrers, was not different to that which occurred in other settings, there was a high number of patient drop-outs: two of the six patients assessed did not continue with treatment after the third week. This might have been because the GPs had referred more complex patients with multiple needs and difficult external circumstances which prevented them from engaging in reflective exploratory work with a student. These drop-outs might also have been the end-product of a primary care culture which places too great an importance on measurable targets, which is more used to shorter interventions, being influenced by the IAPT (Improving Access to Psychological Therapies) programmes, which tend to minimise, or even deny, notions of anxiety and feelings of frailty, fragility, vulnerability and dependence (Rizq, 2012). Additionally, as Launer suggests, accepting psycho-therapists in a general practice 'involves acknowledging in some form that the thinking, working practices, and culture of primary care themselves need help' (Launer et al., 2005, p. 12). Thus the drop-out of these patients might be a symptom of resistance of an established institution to a new development. Placing the Student Psychotherapy Scheme in primary care seemed to cater for a pre-existing need, leaving GPs, nurses and health visitors no longer alone to manage very challenging clinical situations.

TRANSFORMATIONS

Ray Brown and Thanos Tsapas

The most satisfying aspect of running this scheme has been seeing the students develop and mature clinically, academically and personally. It seems that every year the same phenomenon is repeated and this amounts to a transformative experience for both students and teachers. Mezirow defines a transformative experience as 'a process of becoming critically aware of how and why our assumptions have come to constrain the way we perceive, understand, and feel about our world; changing these structures of habitual expectation to make possible a more inclusive, discriminating, and integrating perspective; and finally, making choices or otherwise acting upon these new understandings' (Mezirow, 1991, p. 167). According to this paradigm, the shift results from an exposure in a safe environment to the limitations of one's knowledge, and to the opportunities to reflect on underlying assumptions and to the possibility of alternative approaches.

Clearly the scheme fulfils all this in a unique and creative way. The students have frequently commented that their participation in the scheme was one of the most valuable and rewarding experiences they have had in medical school. They found that the scheme prepared them for their life ahead as doctors, where they sometimes have to deal with extremely challenging situations with limited support. They feel that this experience has strengthened them and allowed them to learn ways to cope better with anxiety and uncertainty. One of the students compared the work of psychotherapy with the work of a surgeon and talked about how the student has to provide his own tools which, although sharpened by preparation and teaching, and further honed in supervision, leave him feeling uncertain and at times inadequate to deal with the emotional wounds of the patient. Fraser and Greenhalgh confirm that 'learning which builds capabilities, takes place when individuals engage with an uncertain and unfamiliar context in a meaningful way. . . . it is reached through a transformative process in which the existing competencies are adapted and tuned to new circumstances. Capability enables one to work effectively in unfamiliar contexts' (Fraser and Greenhalgh, 2001, p. 800).

At the same time, this exposure to uncertainty and unfamiliarity allows students to discover the value of the supervision and also the value of the help they can elicit from their peers. Learning to expose themselves in a safe environment in supervision, to reflect on what they are doing and to allow others to offer them suggestions and further reflections, has continued to be appreciated by students. It also shows them a way to keep themselves healthy and interested in their patients and to increase the satisfaction and enjoyment in their work as students and as future doctors. Through the experience of being supervised they also learn to become more aware of their own limitations and of the importance of asking for help when needed.

The students, in reflecting on their experience of doing psychotherapy, can see that their communication skills have significantly improved. They report that they have not only become better able to listen and empathise with their patients, but they have also found ways to make themselves better understood. They have also learnt to observe and trust their feelings and to use them as tools to understand their patients' internal worlds. This developing capacity for using emotions as tools is experienced by the students as one of the great bonuses of the scheme. The fact that they can then use these ideas to deepen their relationships with their patients, and their peers, fills them with excitement and confidence.

Most students report that they feel empowered by being allowed to become so central to the care of somebody's mind. This is very much in contrast to what one of the students described as the 'handholding comfort' of the undergraduate experience. Others have commented on the difference between the observational, and at times superfluous, role of the student in the UK and the more active participation in patients' care in medical schools in other countries. Students appreciate greatly the commitment they make to their patients and understand how this facilitates the development of a therapeutic relationship. Coupled with this is the importance they learn to place in continuity of care. They are particularly able to appreciate this as they come from clinical placements where short and fragmented interactions with patients are the norm.

Overall the students feel that the scheme has allowed them to greatly enhance their ability to reflect on their practice, which according to Kaufman and Mann (2007) is crucial for life-long self-directed learning, and has also helped them to understand the meaning of being professional, acting with integrity and making their patients their first concern. One student commented on how the scheme offered her a way to understand the journey she had undertaken as medical student. She described how her feelings about the beginning, the middle and the end of the psychotherapy helped her to find parallels with her experience of being a medical student and the professional journey from first-day student to qualified doctor and beyond. She made special reference to the leap of faith that the student has to take when leaving medical school and entering the professional world as a junior doctor.

We think that this leap of faith is the most fundamental process that takes place in the scheme; students are able to move away from thinking only of illness and the body, to whole-person care and to a patient-centred approach.

They are able to take this step without forgetting their roots in biology and science and so manage to widen their practice and enrich their perspectives. The long-lasting effects of the scheme also extend to its supervisors. One of the supervisors in the Bristol scheme participated as a student in the UCL scheme and described how this experience allowed her to restore her confidence in her choice to study medicine after she found out that the everyday practice of medicine focused on illness and not people.

Just as the transformative learning of the students finds a container in the scheme, the scheme itself needs an environment to support and nourish its qualities. As Powell puts it '[the therapeutic group] does not exist in reality outside the special setting in which it takes place, the defined session, the premises in which it is housed and the day or date on which it falls' (Powell, 1989, p. 274). The setting of the Student Psychotherapy Scheme is both the tertiary Psychological Therapies Service or the GP Practice and the University. The scheme feels so full of health and vitality in contrast to much of the NHS, which has been traumatised by threatened closures and job losses, cutbacks and radical changes. It also offers free psychotherapy capacity to local mental health teams, which is greatly valued at times of re-commissioning and strict financial calculations; it has become a point of reflective discussion among local clinicians who have very much welcomed and supported it. In primary care the scheme has offered a valuable resource and an enabling capacity to the local clinicians, helping them to share the burden of patients presenting with complexity and high service usage. Additionally it provides practitioners with a space to which they not only can refer patients, but in which they can also discuss and reflect on their own clinical practice. It also offers psychotherapy expertise, which is usually only found in tertiary services, not in primary care. Finally the scheme has helped to reinforce a culture of continuity and whole-person care which is central to primary care.

For the consultant medical psychotherapist and staff, there is naturally anxiety about supervising inexperienced therapists. We feel that the good functioning and health of the medical student groups coupled with high levels of interest and involvement mitigate against this. Indeed, with this opportunity to revisit psychoanalytic theory and think afresh, we found the work on the scheme enabling and sustaining. We have received feedback from students who have completed the scheme from as far back as 1996. Many have entered careers in psychiatry and general practice. Often they report that the scheme has transformed their interactions with patients, allowing them to have a more human quality, and that participating in it has made them more aware of human complexity.

Acknowledgements

We are indebted to Peter Shoenberg and Jessica Yakeley for the links with the UCL scheme.

Chapter 5

Developing student Balint groups at University College London

Peter Shoenberg and Heather Suckling

Although clinical medical students may confide in each other about their new experiences with patients and are helped by those teachers[1] who are prepared to discuss their emotional reactions to patients and their illnesses as well as to openly consider their patients' feelings, there is usually no regular forum where such a discussion can take place in a safe and nonjudgemental setting. When, as a trainee psychiatrist at University College Hospital, one of us (P.S.) began teaching liaison psychiatry to first-year clinical medical students, he found that they had many anxieties about their role and their experiences with patients that they wanted to share in their small and rather informal group.

History of student Balint groups at UCL

In their first clinical year at UCL, as in many other medical schools, students have special teaching on communication skills and ethical issues and the law, and also have to follow up a cancer patient over several months. In the new UCL curriculum, introduced in 2012, medical students also follow up other patients as part of a new patient pathways module, as well as attending additional seminars on professional practice and writing reflective essays on their clinical experiences.

Around the time that the UCL Student Psychotherapy Scheme began, Michael Balint started two long-term discussion groups, which he referred to as seminars, for medical students to talk about their experiences with patients (Balint, Ball and Hare, 1969). The first was a group for students in the first 6 months of their clinical years and the second was a senior group for students which followed this and lasted until their final year. In his paper about this experience, which lasted for 7 years, Balint made a plea for developing patient-centred rather than illness-centred teaching. Clearly his students got to know their patients very well and were able to discuss their experiences with them at a deep psychological level in this group. For reasons that are not clear, this work with students did not continue.

For a few years after 1998 we received support from the Winnicott and Melanie Klein Trusts and the Academic Department of Psychiatry for three psychoanalysts (Abe Brafman, Fakhri Davids and Ronald Doctor) to run three short-term discussion groups for students attached to the psychiatry firms in their second clinical year. These groups ran for four sessions and they allowed students to reflect on the impact of seeing mentally ill patients. Very important issues were discussed in relation to the students' emotional reactions to being with psychiatric patients (Brafman, 2003), but the leaders and their students were often frustrated by the small number of sessions available to them.

In 2004, when the medical school's annual student intake doubled, we decided to offer the first-year clinical students modified Balint groups (Shoenberg and Suckling, 2004) as an alternative to our Student Psychotherapy Scheme (see Chapter 1). We invited a few of the students, whom we had not been able take onto the Student Psychotherapy Scheme, to participate in a weekly Balint discussion group which met for 1 hour each week for 3 months. Each group began by our asking if any student would like to discuss a patient who had stayed in their mind during the previous week. They were not to rely on notes, but to speak freely about their experience of being with this patient. The other students in the group were then invited to think about and discuss the problem that had been presented. The two leaders interjected only to encourage the students to speak and to facilitate the group process, but did not give the students advice. All that was said in the group was to remain confidential.

We found this experience very rewarding. This development has eventually allowed many more first-year clinical students to benefit from a psycho-therapeutic teaching approach than was previously possible. With the Vice Dean's and the Deputy Director of the medical school's help it has been included on the curriculum as a Student Selected Component (SSC),[2] which generates enough university SIFT (Service Increment for Teaching) funds to pay for two group leaders for each of up to ten groups per year: one is a Balint leader from general practice and the other is a medical psychotherapist from our department. This has the advantage that the Balint leader's expertise in running a Balint group can be shared with the psychotherapist's psycho-dynamic insights into group processes; there is also an advantage in both leaders being medically qualified as this allows for a more accurate identification by the leaders with the students' difficulties.

With the potential of ten groups, up to 100 students can participate each year. Each group now lasts for one and a half hours and each student attends 11 weekly groups. They are then expected to write a reflective essay on a personal experience with a patient discussed in the group and how their thoughts about this have been influenced by this discussion. This fourth-year (first clinical year) student Balint group experience now counts as a final year SSC. The SIFT funding generated by this longitudinal SSC pays for the Balint leaders' work.

The experience of running a student Balint group has proved inspiring and moving, as the students are so enthusiastic, sensitive and imaginative. Sadly, their encounters with their patients, apart from with their cancer patient (as part of the Cancer Patient Pathways programme), are extremely brief, mirroring both the new shorter stays of their patients on the wards and the students' own rapid changes from one medical speciality to another. Often they may only see a patient in groups of two or three students, so that nowadays individual patient encounters are less common.

At the beginning of the first clinical year all students receive a flyer (see Appendix 1) inviting them to a lecture about the UCL Student Psychotherapy Scheme and the student Balint discussion groups. This flyer describes the two schemes and explains that these two schemes will enable them to learn in greater depth about the doctor–patient relationship. At the introductory lecture students are then told more about the two schemes and invited to put their names down at the end of the meeting to be considered for one or other of the schemes. Usually we are able to accommodate all the students asking to join a Balint group, although a proportion drop out before the start of the groups. When the students join a Balint group they are given two hand-outs, one which explains the aims and objectives of the groups and the other which describes the Balint group process and the history of the Balint movement, entitled 'Balint in a Nutshell' (see Appendix 2).

A student Balint group experience

Here is a brief account of a recent student Balint group:

> In our first group, a student, Theo, told us about an 80-year-old woman brought in after collapsing in the street. The junior doctor asked him to clerk the patient, but when he went up to her she angrily told him that she did not want to talk to him. He told the doctor, who insisted he returned to take a history, saying that if he was a junior doctor he would have no choice. He felt it wasn't fair to make this woman speak to him, but decided to do as he was told. On returning he was surprised that she now was willing to see him. As he went through the history he noticed that she couldn't remember what had happened to her and was unaware of what was going on; he thought she might be confused. The group considered the conflict for Theo about doing what the junior doctor wanted rather than following his conscience. Someone said that being rejected by a patient can make you lose your confidence. Melindi said that if she were rejected by a patient, she definitely would not have returned.
>
> Jonathon thought Theo's experience was similar to the experiment where people were made to give electric shocks to somebody and it was found that they too easily followed the dictates of authority rather than the dictates of their conscience. Theo felt that he was only a student and that he had nothing to offer the patient; the others were worried that they were not actually contributing to their patients' care.

In another of the early groups, Jonathon told us about trying to take blood without succeeding. When he offered to try again, the patient said 'get me someone who knows what they are doing'. The registrar told him off, saying that the blood sample was needed urgently, which made him feel guilty. He said that he had never failed to get blood before. It also worried him that he had caused the patient unnecessary pain.

Hanna remembered being helped by a registrar to learn to cannulate a patient. The others agreed that it was better when somebody was there to hold your hand. Others commented that it was all right for a doctor to go on trying but not for them. I said it seemed the discussion was about their fear of hurting the patient versus their fear of being humiliated by the registrar.

As the groups went on the discussions began to focus on the problems of communication: Margaret told us about an elderly woman who had approached her in tears during a tutorial, saying 'do you know that I am dying?' She didn't know how to respond. The junior doctor told her to go back to her bed, but the woman now said that someone had tried to strangle her in the night. After the woman had left, the doctor said he thought this woman was paranoid. Margaret spoke of the contrast between her initial concern, when she had heard the woman saying that she was going to die, and her subsequent feelings when she realised that this woman was confused. Jonathon suggested that as she had been admitted with respiratory distress, her difficulties in breathing might have felt to her as if someone was trying to strangle her. They all felt that the doctor had behaved too dismissively when this woman was so clearly frightened. Arthur said that as students, they were different from the doctors who became de-sensitised when they saw this sort of thing so often, whereas they could still be surprised and shocked by such events.

In another group, Melindi spoke about an elderly Tamil woman who was calling for help for her pain. The first time she saw her, she felt influenced by the nurses who told her not to get involved because this woman complained too much. However, the next day she learned on the ward round that this woman had had a colonoscopy and that her bowel had been perforated. Now she felt badly about her initial dismissive reaction towards her and returned to talk to her. The woman spoke Tamil, which she couldn't speak but she realised that she might understand Hindi which was her language. However, the woman's voice was very indistinct, so it was hard for Melindi to work out what she said: she often had to repeat phrases to make herself understood. The patient told her that she wanted to be helped back into bed. She called a nurse who said she would have to get a hoist for her. She waited with the woman, keeping a conversation going, and eventually she returned to the nurses' station where she found the nurses talking. They said they would come, but they still didn't come to help her for some time. Melindi felt upset about the whole experience, particularly when she learned that this woman had developed necrosis of her bowel and that the surgical team were worried about her condition. The woman said she thought they were all liars.

I wondered why they thought the nurses had taken against this woman. Arthur said he thought the language barrier was an issue and then Jonathon said that if the woman had been white and middle class she might have got some attention. Hanna described a patient whose children were a lawyer and a doctor where the nurses behaved differently. In fact Melindi noticed that the nurse behaved in a better way towards the woman when she had thought that Melindi was a relative; then the nurse changed back to her old manner when she realised that Melindi was a medical student. The group were shocked. Tahir talked about a report about the mistreatment of elderly patients in hospital and wondered if this woman's age had contributed to her neglect by the nurses. She hadn't wanted to eat any of the food she was given; Melindi had offered to go to a nearby Indian restaurant to get food for her but she had refused. The other Balint leader wondered if in fact she had become this woman's advocate. He thought this woman must have been very angry about what had been done to her by the surgeons. Tahir said that people from his part of the world took such events in a different way from Westerners.

In another group the shy and usually silent student Arthur presented a middle-aged man with chronic heart disease, who had welcomed him, saying that he was glad to help students to learn something. He talked of his life before he had become ill: he was a keen sportsman and seemed to be coping with his illness with a positive attitude. Arthur, a keen footballer, who was wearing an Arsenal supporters' shirt in our group, had clearly identified with him. Then, as the man talked about his family, he burst into tears speaking of his son who had died at a young age. Arthur didn't know how to handle this situation: he had been told that if a patient became very emotional, the student should not do anything to make the situation worse. He asked the group what they would have done, as he had felt reluctant to ask more questions for fear of spoiling the man's positive attitude. Some students felt that he shouldn't make the man more upset by probing into the story of the death: one said he couldn't imagine what it would be like to experience the death of a child. Two other students said that it might have been worth asking this man if he wanted to talk about his son. They spoke of the pressure they were under to produce a good medical history, as opposed to feeling they could spend time listening to the emotions of their patients.

Arthur subsequently wrote in his reflective essay:

When the majority of the group seemed not necessarily to agree with what I had done I felt defensive, feeling that if they had been in front of him they would have acted similarly, but then I saw my patient two days later. He joked with me saying, 'I'm invisible, I've been discharged'. I realised there was a strong bond between us and thought of the comment by one of the Balint leaders that as a young man I might have connected with him, as he might have seen me as having similarities to the son he had lost. This allowed me to interact with him at a more meaningful and personal level. I realised he was interested in my education and my love of football. Now I think about my hesitation to speak about his loss when he got so upset, I can see that by simply asking whether a patient wishes to talk more about an issue means you give yourself the possibility of learning more about the patient on a more personal level while giving the patient the power to make the decision about where the consultation is going.

(Shoenberg, 2012)

Common themes in Balint groups

The Balint groups provide the students with an opportunity to explore a number of themes. We found in the first Balint group we conducted (Shoenberg and Suckling, 2004) that initially the students briefly discussed several cases in the early sessions and that much time was spent on general issues, but as the students became more confident they began to discuss individual cases in greater depth. Often in the early groups students spoke about their anxiety that they had no real role and of their concern that they were exploiting the patients in order to learn to become doctors. Later they began to explore their communications with patients in a more positive way and to appreciate their value to their patients.

Suckling reviewed three consecutive groups that we had conducted, recording a total of 63 cases as having been discussed. She identified 17 themes, of which the following ten were most common:

1   The student's role: Students often spoke of incidents where they felt they were in the way, for example, when a seriously ill patient was being assessed by a doctor and there was no role for the student. However, there were other occasions when the student was given specific tasks to do and then he or she felt a useful member of the team. Students often felt 'at the mercy of the patient':

One student described his first attempt at taking a medical history. As he approached the patient ready to ask her permission, she suddenly said: 'No! I said no to the students yesterday, I say no today and I'll say no tomorrow, I will not speak to students!' The group laughed with him, but they realised how upsetting it was for him to be rejected in this way. Later, they began to consider the situation from the patient's point of view and wondered if perhaps she had not been feeling well or whether many other students had approached her that day.

2   Confidentiality: Students spoke of being taught about the need for privacy when talking to patients:

> One student wondered how they should have taken a history of constipation from an elderly patient, who was hard of hearing, on an open ward with only a curtain to separate him from the other patients.

> Another student spoke of a patient who admitted exaggerating his symptoms, by telling the doctors she was suicidal, in order to gain admission. She was an alcoholic who hoped to get inpatient detoxification by this means, because she knew that otherwise she would only be offered outpatient treatment. The student wondered if he should tell the doctors or collude with the patient.

3   Consent: There were several experiences of difficulties about informed consent:

> An elderly woman was admitted because of rectal bleeding, whom the student felt was being coerced by her relative. She had been very co-operative and the student felt that she had taken a good history. However, when the patient's son joined them, he had told her that his mother was demented and her problem was in fact a cancer. He added that his mother did not want conventional treatment but preferred herbal remedies. When the student later saw the patient alone, he found that she would like to have any treatment that would help, including the recommended chemotherapy. However, when the doctor saw the patient, the son said firmly that his mother had made it clear that she did not want treatment. The student was able to explain her concern to the doctor who promised to consult the patient without her son.

4   The very ill patient: Students described concerns about how to approach a seriously ill patient and how to answer their questions. This could be difficult if one did not know how much the patient knew, or what to say if their condition was very serious:

> A student approached a patient, having read that he was awaiting surgery for a pancreatic tumour; but after having taken his history the

patient had told him that he had already undergone surgery and knew he had an inoperable gall bladder cancer. Although the student had prepared himself for the possibility that he had a serious illness, he was shocked to find that the patient already knew the bad news and he did not know how to react. He told the group that he had wanted to run away, but he did stay with him and was amazed at how he helped him to speak of other things.

5   Death and dying: The students were aware of the risk of being completely detached from the patient's and their own emotions in the effort to remain 'professional'. Sometimes they saw this reflected in doctors' behaviour:

> A student was in Casualty when a 50-year-old woman was brought in after taking cocaine, swallowing bleach and then jumping from the fifth floor of a building. While being treated for her severe injuries her heart stopped and the student was asked to do the cardiac compressions, for the first time in her training. However, the patient died soon afterwards and the doctors just stated that she was dead. To her horror the whole team moved on to the next case, with no discussion or attempt to ask her how she was feeling, leaving her alone with the dead patient. She wondered if the patient's history had influenced the doctors' behaviour. The group asked her how she had coped: she said that when she got home she had spoken to a friend who reassured her that she had done her best to help this patient.

6   Revulsion towards patients: Students talked about coping with their feelings of revulsion on seeing some patients, either because of disfigurement or poor personal hygiene or because of prejudices demonstrated by the patient:

> A student spoke of having been shocked by seeing a woman with a terrible facial disfigurement. She needed to take a history from her and as she was with her husband, she said she would have preferred to speak to him rather than the patient. However, she managed to overcome her horror and had spoken directly to her. To her surprise she found that when she began to speak to her she did not even notice her disfigurement.

7   History taking: Many difficulties with history taking came up. It might not be possible to find a patient willing to be seen by a student, or because students were asked to see patients in pairs, it was easier to cover a full history, but more difficult to speak about sensitive issues in the presence of the other student. Sometimes it was difficult to believe the patient's story:

One young woman had severe abdominal pain, but was a known drug addict whom the staff did not trust. The student was worried that she might be in genuine pain and was troubled as she kept on asking her to get her more morphine.

The commonest difficulty experienced was the conflict between trying to listen to the patient's own story and taking a full systematic history with the standard questions. How could they get silent patients to speak, or garrulous ones to stop talking or cope with patients who denied or exaggerated their symptoms?

8   Professional boundaries (see Chapter 6): Did one behave like a professional and risk being impersonal or like a friend when it was easy to be over familiar? The students found it particularly difficult to relate to patients of similar ages to their own, especially those of the opposite sex. How did you examine patients whom you might find attractive, or who found the student attractive? Issues about touching patients were often mentioned:

Shortly after a terrorist attack in London, patients who had come to the hospital with minor injuries were asked to remain there for 3 hours after treatment to ensure that more serious injuries did not go undiagnosed and to allow them time to recover from shock. A student was allocated to each patient to look after them, fetch refreshments, help them arrange transport home and make sure they were interviewed by the police. One student in the group had been allocated a young lawyer dressed in a formal suit, who had told her that he was 'absolutely fine' and had wanted to leave. Initially she felt intimidated but she realised that his denial was probably due to shock. After a time he began to tell her about his job as a senior member of a city law firm. He had just begun this job and was still living more than a hundred miles away so he realised he was going to have difficulty in getting home because of the serious disruption to all transport in London. He allowed the student to help him and gradually his defences fell away, so that by the time he left he looked very sad although he was very appreciative. The student told the group that she had wanted to give him a hug, but she had felt it would be unprofessional. When a group member said that perhaps it was she who had needed a hug after such an emotional experience, she smiled and said that when she did leave the hospital she had met an old friend who had given her a hug.

9   The student–patient relationship: Students recognised the privilege of being able to enter the patients' lives and share some of their experiences and they were surprised how some patients were able to trust them even

though they were not yet doctors. They often felt that they were giving nothing to the patient and were a nuisance, but an appreciative patient could help them to feel valued.

10   Doctors' attitudes and communication: Students were often impressed by the doctors' respect for patients but also they reported feeling uncomfortable with the position of power that the doctors held, e.g. doctors' approaches to clinical teaching and their good and bad communication with staff, relatives and patients. They were impressed by the doctors' respect for those patients who might have aroused feelings of revulsion, but also disturbed by some doctors' difficulties in coping with death. Sometimes they felt patients were being stereotyped:

> A student was working on a surgical ward where the junior doctor advised him not to clerk the patient in the single room because he was 'psychotic' (he had tried to commit suicide by throwing himself in front of a train). At this stage in his training the student had no experience of psychiatry and had assumed that the patient might be dangerous. One day the ward was very busy and the doctor had asked this student to take blood from this patient for tests. He entered the room with trepidation, but the patient had smiled at him. When he tried to straighten the patient's arm it clearly caused pain and the student had been frightened that he would react violently; however, he had just extended his other arm and as the student bent over him to take the blood, the patient had said 'you smell really nice'. One of the group members asked the presenter if he thought the patient found him attractive, but he said that was not his concern: he had been thinking of Hannibal Lecter in *The Silence of the Lambs*! However, afterwards the patient had been really appreciative and thanked the student for talking to him, saying as he left, 'You are a fantastic nurse.'

Other themes commonly discussed in Balint groups were anger in patients, doctors and students, frustration, dealing with distressed patients, denial, problems about the quality of life of patients, diagnoses, and challenging assumptions (Suckling, 2005).[3]

The students in this study also gave us feedback that participating in the group had increased their confidence, improved their communication skills, encouraged whole-patient medicine and reflection, while providing support and increasing their enjoyment of their work (Suckling, 2005).

Some of the difficulties in running groups

1   Student anxieties about speaking: Often in the early groups students are unsure about speaking in such a personal and revealing way about their feelings for patients in front of peers, many of whom they may hardly

know. It is important for the leaders to be as encouraging as possible. Students may fear that they themselves are in some way being analysed or judged by the leaders. It is important to emphasise that what is said in the group is confidential. In spite of all the encouragement to speak, some students remain rather quiet and do not participate a great deal in the discussions. As the group members become more confident with each other, the chances of all the members participating, increases. There is a definite advantage to having a minimum of 11 group sessions.

2   Problems about attendance: In anticipation of this, we like to interview all the students who have put their names down for a group. This allows us to set out the aims and objectives of the groups (see Appendices 2 and 3), to emphasise the importance of the students bringing their own clinical experiences to the group and of regular attendance, and to deal with any queries about this scheme. Because the Balint group is now an SSC, students are expected to attend regularly in order to pass this SSC; the mandatory reflective essay, to be written by each student at the end of the group, is an additional motivating factor.

3   Group size: If a group has too few students in it, the absence of two students can affect the quality of the group interaction. On the other hand, too many students can make the group unwieldy and inhibit students from speaking. Ideally there should be ten students in each group.

4   Ensuring that all the students present a patient: It may be a problem to get each student to present at least one patient whom they have got to know in greater depth, and to consider their feelings about their relationship with this patient. Although the most natural patient for them to present is the cancer patient whom they follow up during their first clinical year (as part of the Cancer Patient Pathway programme), we encourage them to bring clinical experiences of patients they have seen on the wards or in the outpatient clinic. Balint emphasised that it is the interaction between the doctor (or student) and his or her patient that is crucial for understanding the patient. However, students often prefer the less threatening option of reporting clinical situations witnessed, in which someone else (usually a doctor or a nurse) has related to a patient in a way that has concerned or disturbed them. While it is important to allow such discussions to take place, particularly in the early groups, these should not be at the expense of student discussions about direct contact with their own patients.

5   Ethical issues: The students sometimes present cases where the doctor's behaviour has made them feel uncomfortable, and they felt he or she had not acted in accordance with ethical guidelines. There is sometimes a tension between respect for patients and the perceived learning needs of the student.

(a) Examinations without consent: There are strict guidelines for students about carrying out intimate examinations on patients who are under anaesthetic. They are required to obtain written consent from the patient before he or she goes to theatre.

In one group a student described how the surgeon told him to do a rectal examination on an anaesthetised patient. The student did not know the patient and had no permission from him to do this, but he felt pressurised by the consultant who implied that the student did not want to learn. He went ahead and did the rectal examination but felt badly about it, and in the group he said, 'I hope in future I will have the courage to refuse.' It transpired that other students had been faced with similar dilemmas. The problem is exacerbated by the fact that the consultant is often involved in the assessment of that student.

(b) Examining patients without capacity:

A student, Mary, described how she had been told to examine an elderly patient who had memory loss after a stroke. She was repeatedly asking for her daughter and weeping. Although her daughter saw her frequently she could not remember her. Mary was reluctant to examine her as the patient was clearly distressed and could not give consent, but the doctor insisted, because 'she has good signs'. Mary did examine her, but 'felt awful' as she felt she had taken advantage of a vulnerable patient who was already upset.

(c) Should students report doctors' unethical behaviour?

A learning-disabled woman with severe physical disabilities was in theatre, anaesthetised and needing to be catheterised. This proved difficult: two registrars had tried without success and so then they had asked for help, but even the consultant they approached had failed. Another consultant ridiculed them and said he would photograph their attempts and put the image on a hospital website.

The student who reported the story was horrified, especially as he felt that the patient could have been identified, but did not think the doctor would carry out his threat. However, the doctor did photograph them attempting the catheterisation on the naked anaesthetised patient; yet no one in the theatre said anything. The students in the group were shocked, and someone in the group wondered whether such a thing would have occurred if the patient had not had a learning disability. There was a prolonged silence. Then one of the group asked what could be done.

The medical school did have a procedure for reporting such things anonymously, but at the time the students did not really trust it. One student said, 'How can it remain anonymous if the incident is investigated?' Another said, 'There is huge anxiety that if you challenge a senior doctor you will jeopardise your career.' Another said, 'Surely if you do not report it, you are condoning it?' There was a useful discussion, after which it was agreed that the leaders, with the students' permission, would report the incident anonymously. As a result of this and also because of concerns raised by other students, a Raising Concerns Website was developed for the medical students.

This encourages students first of all to discuss the matter with a trusted senior or their personal tutor, but if the issue is not resolved in this way, they can report it to the medical school anonymously and their anonymity will be respected. However, at this point, it is explained to them that, in order that for there to be a formal investigation, they may be asked to give their names. They are told that they are not obliged to do so, but if they do give their names they will be properly supported. In this case the leaders were able to report back to the students that this website had been developed. The original incident was subsequently discussed with the perpetrator privately by a very senior medical member of the medical school. Now all students are told about the website.

6   Vulnerable students: Occasionally a vulnerable student may join the group in the hope of getting help for their own problems; very rarely a student has brought up personal issues which are clearly beyond the scope of the group. In this event we offer to speak with the student outside the group and if necessary help them to find appropriate psychological help.

Student Balint groups in other countries

Student Balint groups have been used in several countries, including Germany (Drees and Schwartz, 1990), Austria (Sollner et al., 1992), Italy (Castiglioni and Bellini, 1982), Switzerland (Luban-Plozza, 1995; 1989), Poland (Jugowar and Skommer, 2003), Finland (Torppa et al., 2008), South Africa (Levenstein, 1980), the United States (Brazeau et al., 1998; Turner, 2005), Australia (Parker and Leggett, 2012), Brazil (Taveira et al., 2010) and Peru (Mendoza, 2009). In Germany many medical schools now have student Balint groups, some of which are mixed groups involving students and doctors together as participants. A variant on Balint groups introduced by Schuffel (1983) in Germany is called Anamnesegruppen in which there is a focus on the case history of an individual patient and the difficulties experienced by the student in making emotional contact with their patient. There are also groups organised by the medical students to consider patient-oriented learning (Otten, personal communication, 2012).

The International Balint Federation now makes a biannual award called the Ascona Prize for essays by medical students reflecting on their experience of a significant relationship to a patient.

Conclusion

Whereas running a Student Psychotherapy Scheme requires considerable resources, as well as complex clinical governance and raises ethical issues, and is only available to a few students, Balint group teaching, which also requires experienced group leaders, can accommodate many more students because of its shorter duration and its group approach. As a Student Selected Component it can be included in the curriculum and so also generates university funds that pay for the Balint leaders it requires.

Balint wanted all the first-year clinical students to have the experience of participating in an initial 6-month group. We suspect that if such teaching became obligatory for all students, rather than an option, some of the aliveness and imaginative quality of the groups would go, but there could be an enormous value in offering some students the chance to be in a group for 6 months or in the opportunity of being in another Balint group later in their training.

We see in these groups how students begin to see themselves as future doctors with a responsibility for another person. In this process they change from feeling they are mere observers, of little use to their patients, to realising that their listening and caring skills are at a premium; this is often in settings where they turn out to be the only person with enough time to consider the emotional aspects of the patient's illness. The Balint group experience helps them to appreciate the significance of emotions in medical illness and with that to appreciate their true value as students for their patients.

Notes

1   One GP teacher (John Horder), rather than asking his student what the diagnosis was, asked what he or she had felt about the consultation they had just observed.
2   SSCs are optional modules within the undergraduate medical syllabus in UK medical schools. In 2003 the GMC required that between 25% and 33% of curricular time be available for SSCs.
3   A qualitative study by Torppa et al., of a smaller number of consecutive sessions of two student Balint groups (15 sessions) found similar themes emerging: feelings related to patients, building professional identity, negative role models, cooperation with other medical professionals, witnessing injustice, value conflicts, difficult human relationships, incurable patients and role confusion) (Torppa et al., 2008).

Appendix I

UCL MEDICAL SCHOOL

DEPARTMENT OF MENTAL HEALTH SCIENCES

LEARNING ABOUT THE CLINICAL STUDENT–PATIENT RELATIONSHIP

THE BEGINNINGS OF THE DOCTOR–PATIENT RELATIONSHIP IN PRACTICE

NOTICE FOR FIRST CLINICAL YEAR (YEAR 4) MEDICAL STUDENTS

RE THE STUDENT PSYCHOTHERAPY SCHEME & STUDENT 'BALINT' DISCUSSION GROUPS AT UCL.

BOTH SCHEMES ARE OFFERED AS STUDENT SELECTED COMPONENTS (SSCs)

I Student Psychotherapy Scheme

Medical students in the first clinical year may take on for once-weekly individual psychotherapy a patient attending the Outpatient Department of Psychotherapy. This psychotherapy is supervised by one of the members of the department and has been a very popular scheme both in the past and the present. This enables medical students to learn more about the doctor–patient relationship, as well as how to work in a psychotherapeutic way with patients.

The scheme has now been operating for 50 years and allows up to 15 medical students to take part each year. Each student sees a patient, who has been carefully selected for individual psychotherapy, each week for an hour and discusses the session in a psychotherapy supervision group consisting of four to five students with a group supervisor. There are currently a number of groups and some vacancies will be shortly arising.

2 Student clinical discussion (Balint) groups

Alternatively, we also offer students the chance to join a weekly discussion group, lasting for 11 weeks, to talk about their clinical experiences with patients and to explore the emotional aspects of illness and to learn more about the doctor–patient (student–patient) relationship. These groups, which are based on the ideas of Michael Balint, start at the beginning of January and the beginning of May. Each of the groups is taken by two specialist leaders, one of whom is a psychotherapist and one of whom is a general practitioner. The groups have also proved to be very popular. There will be five or six groups with vacancies for up to 60 students. The groups last for one and a half hours each week and are held at 5.30pm on a weekday. This is recognised as an SSC which is completed by writing a reflective essay based on the group discussions. This will integrate with and enhance the existing requirement for students to follow the progress of a cancer patient by offering supportive reflection on the psychological factors involved in this relationship. Reflection in depth on other patients encountered in clinical work will also be encouraged. These groups promote students' professionalism in this area which is of fundamental importance to any medical or surgical specialty.

To take part in either scheme to fulfil your SSC you should attend this talk

Note that students doing these SSCs will be allowed time off in their final year after exams corresponding to the time devoted – the equivalent of four weeks

To find out more about these options please come to the meeting on Wednesday 18th September 2013 at 3.00pm

Venue: Lecture Theatre 1, Cruciform Building

Appendix 2

BALINT GROUPS for MEDICAL STUDENTS
(Handout for Balint group students)

AIMS AND LEARNING OUTCOMES

Aims of the Group Sessions:
1   To provide the students with an opportunity to explore the emotional aspects of their work in a safe environment
2   To increase the students' understanding of their patients' communication
3   To provide support and supervision* for the students
4   To encourage the students to reflect on their work

Learning Outcomes:

After the course the students will:
1   Be able to consider their clinical encounters in a new light
2   Become aware of the significance of the relationship between the doctor/ student and the patient
3   Be able to recognise the feelings which are evoked by the interaction with the patient and be able to use these for the benefit of the patient
4   Be able to use the group to express and process anxieties and frustrations about their work
5   Recognise the inherent value of the consultation itself
6   Become aware of their own limitations
7   Value their own humanity and personality and the effects of these on the patient

*supervision in the psychotherapeutic sense

BALINT IN A NUTSHELL
(Handout for Balint group students)

History of the Balint group
- The name is that of Michael Balint, a Hungarian psychoanalyst.
- His main work was as a psychoanalyst at the Tavistock Clinic, in London.
- He started groups for GPs in the 1950s to study the doctor–patient relationship, he described them as 'Training-cum-research' groups.
- He worked closely, and ran groups with his third wife, Enid – a social worker and marriage guidance counsellor. Her influence on medical training is probably as great as his.

N.B. Michael Balint ran a Balint group for medical students at University College Hospital in the late 1960s.

What is a 'traditional' Balint group?
- It consists of six to twelve doctors (or students) with one or two leaders and it meets regularly.
- Meetings usually last for one to two hours and the group continues for one or more years.
- The method is that of case presentation without notes.

What happens in a Balint group?
- The leader asks 'Who has a case?'
- The presenter who volunteers tells the story of a consultation: this is not a standard case presentation, but a description of what happened between the doctor/student and the patient.
- It need not be long, complicated or exciting but something that is continuing to occupy the presenter's mind. It may be puzzling, or has left the presenter feeling angry, frustrated, irritated or sad.
- The group discusses the relationship between the doctor/student and patient and tries to understand what is happening that evokes these feelings.
- The feelings which the patient evokes are significant and may be reflected in the presenter or in the group. This can help us to understand the patient.
- All discussions within the group are confidential.

What can a Balint group do?
- It provides an opportunity for you to reflect on your work.
- It can provide an outlet for anxieties and frustrations generated by your work.
- It can arouse your interest in a patient whom you have previously found upsetting, annoying or 'difficult'.
- It can open your mind to other possibilities, both of diagnosis and day-to-day management.

- The group provides support and improves communication with patients and other professionals.
- It can improve your job satisfaction and the patient's perception of care.

What does a Balint group not do?
- It does not tell you 'how to do' things.
- It does not provide easy answers.
- It will not solve all your problems with patients.

Who was Michael Balint?
- He was born in Budapest in 1896, the son of a GP.
- He became interested in psychoanalysis after first hearing Freud speak in 1918 and when he met his first wife, Alice, who was a psychoanalyst.
- He obtained his doctorate in medicine in 1920 and initially worked as a biochemist.
- Later he undertook psychoanalytic training in Budapest; his analyst was Sandor Ferenczi.
- Balint worked as a psychoanalyst in Budapest during the Fascist regime, but in 1939 came to Manchester (UK) as a refugee.
- In 1945 he was appointed as a psychoanalyst at the Tavistock Clinic.
- In the early 1950s he began his work with GPs – the Balint group was born.
- In 1957 *The Doctor, his Patient and the Illness*, his seminal work, was published.
- The founders of the Royal College of General Practitioners were profoundly influenced by Balint's ideas; they formed the basis of modern postgraduate training for general practice.
- It was because of his influence that small group work forms an essential part of GP training.
- He used the term 'patient-centred medicine' in his description of the group he ran at University College Hospital for medical students in 1969.

Perhaps the essence of Balint groups has always been to share experiences and enable people to observe and rethink aspects of their relationships with patients and their work as doctors.

(from Balint et al., 1993, *The Doctor, the Patient and the Group*)

Useful websites:
The Balint Society: www.balint.co.uk
The International Balint Federation: www.balintinternational.com

Chapter 6

Professional identity and confusion of boundaries

Sotiris Zalidis

Introduction

First-year clinical medical students are at a crucial point in the development of their professional identity. Because less time separates them from lay persons than hospital consultants they tend to identify more easily with patients, particularly when they are similar in age to the student. Also the students have just started coming into contact with seriously ill patients who are in the grip of powerful feelings. Such feelings may be experienced by the students as intrusive and overwhelming and may threaten their sense of self and emerging professional identity. Medical students can easily become emotionally detached because the default setting in the culture of medical education is affective distance and clinical neutrality. Emotional detachment may seem a tempting solution because, at least, not feeling anything will protect against emotional responses that are too complicated or distressing for the learner. Students are on the lookout for role models so they are quick to notice any negative emotions of hostility, indifference, frustration and impatience that their supervisors express, as well as the positive emotions of caring, compassion and kindness shown by them towards patients (Shapiro, 2011). Their professional identity is likely to be shaped by these role models.

Professional identity and role models

It has been shown that medical students' interpersonal skills with patients decline as their medical education progresses (Helfer, 1970). This is particularly true for the students' ability to take a good social history. It seems that as students learn more about the science of medicine, they find it harder simply to talk with patients, and may come to devalue this kind of activity. What have been easy exchanges during the first years later become an awkward and unproductive series of closed questions. Another study found that as training progresses students seem to lose their grasp of the patient's total health picture and focus more and more on biomedical issues (Martin et al., 1976). It seems that in their early years of medical school, students do a better job of talking with patients than fully trained doctors.

Medical educators have taken on board the criticism that the emphasis on basic science in the curriculum was out of proportion to its relevance to clinical practice and introduced communication skills training, which is now an important part of the medical curriculum. However, despite the introduction of communication skills teaching, a recent survey of medical students' attitudes to mental and medical illnesses (Korszun et al., 2012) found that attitudes towards patients with unexplained abdominal symptoms were clearly worse in senior than in junior students. The authors concluded that students probably acquired their negative attitudes from doctors using pejorative terms such as 'heart sink' to describe patients whose frustrating symptoms and personalities could not be understood and controlled easily using a conventional biomedical model. Hafferty has written about aspects of the hidden curriculum which influences student attitudes (Hafferty, 1998).

However, there has been some interesting research suggesting that students' and doctors' attitudes to patients can be improved by certain teaching interventions. In a study by a group of Israeli investigators that targeted personal skills of emotional self-awareness and sensitivity to patients (Kramer et al., 1987), Israeli medical students and their medical teachers participated over 5 weeks in ten 90-minute twice-weekly sessions on interviewing skills. In these meetings the students talked about admitting a patient to the hospital, diagnosing a life-threatening disease, death and dying, teamwork, uncertainty and chronic disease. In addition, time was taken for role play in which the students and their teachers played the role of patients, doctors and family members. The students' and doctors' rejecting behaviour, in their visits with real patients, was studied both before and after this training: rejecting behaviour included sarcasm, contempt, verbal rejection, non-responsiveness to the patient's statements, and avoiding eye contact.

The results were fascinating: before training, the medical students engaged in much less rejecting behaviour than the doctors. Students averaged about six negative behaviours per interview before training, while doctors averaged almost twice as many. One year after training, students engaged in two rejecting behaviours per interview on average, as compared to the doctors' five. A control group of students who had not received this training averaged 11 rejecting behaviours per interview. Thus negativity was substantially lower for both medical students and doctors at 1 year after the teaching intervention, while members of the control group increased their rejecting behaviours over the same time. The study underscores the damage that doctors may do as role models to their students. Medical students imitate their clinical teachers' patterns of dealing with patients. If teachers exhibit a dehumanised and rejecting pattern of communication with patients, students will learn that pattern. This study suggests that damage done to young medical students' ability and inclination to be compassionate and empathic may be prevented, diminished and undone. It is also reassuring to see that even well-respected and established doctors can be made to change longstanding patterns of communication for the better (Roter and Hall, 2006).

Changing attitudes

In the UK, Michael and Enid Balint's research has provided medical education with a unique instrument for helping doctors and students understand their own emotional responses and the emotions of their patients, by discussing their encounters with patients in the safe environment of a well-led group. The ability to understand our own feelings and the feelings of the other, and to act so as to shape our feelings to make them easier to bear, is central to handling relationships. All rapport, which is at the root of caring, stems from a capacity for empathy (Zalidis, 2001).

What is empathy?

The term empathy was coined in 1909 by a British psychologist, E. B. Titchener. He considered that empathy stems from a physical imitation of the distress of another, which includes an unconscious imitation of his facial expression, which then evokes feelings in us. Titchener (1909) distinguished empathy from sympathy, which recognises the plight of another, but does not include sharing the other's feelings. Empathy in other words is possible because emotions are communicable. A person in the grip of an emotion broadcasts it and we observers resonate with his transmission. The contagious quality of the broadcast drags the observer into resonance. Its intensity is decreased to the extent that the broadcaster or the receiver learns to modulate his display of the emotion.

Empathy builds on emotional self-awareness. The more open we are to our emotions, the more skilled we are in reading the feelings of others. Mature empathy is the ability to enter imaginatively and accurately into the thoughts, feelings, hopes and fears of another person. This ability to stand in somebody else's shoes and allow them to do the same to us is a developmental achievement and a sign of health. It also depends on the capacity for self-control of our anger, distress or excitement and restraint of the impulse to express feelings in immediate action: this is achieved by learning to pause to reflect upon what we are feeling and why we are having particular feelings.

Learning to handle the emotions of the other: Balint groups as a form of empathic exercise

Because 90% of an emotional message is non-verbal, the key to the intuition of another's feelings is the ability to read non-verbal information such as the tone of voice, gesture, facial expressions, and so on. Messages such as anxiety in someone's tone of voice or irritation in the quickness of a gesture are almost always taken in unconsciously and responded to without necessarily being aware that emotional communication has taken place. We share the affect just triggered in the other person to the extent that we mimic the operation of the same muscle groups. Some doctors can resonate more easily than others with the emotions of their patients. When this capacity is not understood, however, it may feel like a burden. Individuals may be vulnerable to empathic over-arousal: Hoffman (2000) defines this as an involuntary process that occurs when an observer's distress becomes so painful and intolerable that it is transformed into intense personal distress that can impair empathy. If we resonate easily with the affect of our patients we have to develop a way of filtering or modulating the intensity of our emotional response. Balint groups can help students to learn how to contain the emotions aroused in clinical encounters by helping them during group discussions to develop reflective self-awareness and become acquainted with their emotions. In these groups the leaders sometimes invite the participants to put themselves into the shoes of the patient who has been presented and sometimes into those of the presenting student and imagine their feelings and their relationships. Such group work is a form of empathic exercise.

Balint groups with first-year clinical medical students

When Michael Balint and his colleagues published their paper on *Training Medical Students in Patient-centred Medicine* in 1969 (Balint et al., 1969) it was based on seminars that had been running at UCH for 7 years. At that time medical services were organised differently and it was possible for students to follow up in the outpatient department certain patients they had met on the ward, after their discharge. Balint had set out to explore questions such as:

1   Whether patient-centred medicine could lead to a better understanding of the illness of the patient.
2   What kind of help could students be expected to give to their patients when they adopted this approach.
3   What demands could the seminar make on the students and they on themselves.
4   What kind of training could be offered to the students to help their patients in this different way.

The concept of patient-centred medicine was created in contrast with illness-centred medicine. It aimed to arrive at an overall diagnosis that while including full consideration of the underlying organic disease, allowed for consideration of the illness as a meaningful phase in a person's life history. One of the difficulties Balint and his colleagues encountered was the students' uneasiness about exploring personal areas of the patient's life, which some considered would infringe the patient's privacy. Those who persisted discovered that their difficulties about this issue were mainly subjective and quickly disappeared when they acquired a technique of 'sympathetic objectivity' described by Balint. The students who adopted this technique found that their patients were relieved to talk about their personal life, and that their clinical encounter had been a satisfying experience. Balint realised that there were differences among the students in their attitude to emotional problems and in their capacity to create a sufficiently comfortable atmosphere that allowed the patient to talk. He doubted whether all students could learn the skills required for this type of work.

The medical landscape has changed considerably since Balint's time. It has become almost impossible for students to follow up patients, because their teaching attachments are so short. The only opportunity for observation of continuity of care at UCL (apart from the UCL Student Psychotherapy Scheme) is the project which involves following up, over five visits, a cancer patient (Cancer Patient Pathways Project). Since 2004, first-year clinical medical students at UCL are offered modified student Balint discussion groups for 11 one-and-a-half-hour-long weekly sessions in which they can present and discuss encounters with patients that have left an emotional trace in the student. The emphasis in these groups is on helping the student to increase his awareness of patients' emotions and to enhance his or her own reflective self-awareness. In this way we hope to give these students a deeper understanding of the doctor–patient relationship.

When I started co-leading these Balint groups we encouraged the students to report emotions aroused during a personal interaction with a patient, thus replicating the method of Balint groups for general practitioners. However, we found that students frequently presented 'situations', rather than personal interactions with patients, such as their observations of interactions between health care professionals and patients that had affronted the student's ideal of doctor–patient relationship. The discrepancy between their ideal of a doctor and the actual doctor had often left the student perplexed and sometimes traumatised. The students felt that they needed an opportunity to share this disillusionment in the Balint group. The ensuing discussion in the Balint group allowed the students to think more carefully about their identifications with their teachers, which helped them to learn about how to form their own professional identity.

Four examples of patients discussed by students in Balint groups

Since 2011 the students have been required to write a reflective essay at the end of their 11 sessions in the group. Here they must give an account of an encounter with a patient and how their subsequent discussion about this in the group changed their thoughts about it. The summaries of the four essays that follow illustrate the range of emotions that clinical medical students may have to deal with in their daily experiences with patients.

Learning about professional boundaries

One of the few opportunities to follow up a patient over a period of several months is provided by the Cancer Patient Pathways Project. Its stated aim is to increase the students' understanding of oncology. All the students are expected to meet a cancer patient and follow him or her up over five visits either at the hospital or outside.

In her essay, one of our medical students wrote movingly about the help she got from the discussion at the Balint group for her distressing and disconcerting experiences that had overwhelmed her. The patient, a middle-aged married woman, had become terminally ill and had been admitted to a hospice. The student wanted to experience this new environment and asked whether she could visit her there. She was shocked, however, to discover how ill the patient looked and how upset her relatives were. The patient's mother started crying and the student became acutely aware of just how terribly sad and desperate the situation really was. She felt identified with the patient's relatives and after a couple of hours of talking by her bedside, the patient's husband offered her a lift to the train station in his car. As it was raining heavily she accepted. When they arrived at the station, the husband started crying and the student felt out of her depth in this unfamiliar situation and unsure of how to proceed. She also started crying. After a little while they both began to compose themselves, but the student was so upset by the experience that she took the wrong train and did not realise she was going in the wrong direction until an hour had elapsed.

The Balint discussion helped her realise that part of her discomfort was not because of any failure on her part to meet her patient's expectations, but rather was the result of her poorly defined role. Was she acting like a medical student or a friend? Who was the patient? Was the patient the cancer sufferer, her mother or her husband? Being outside the hospital and in the husband's car had blurred the professional boundaries and placed her in a position of uncertainty and unfamiliarity.

The student was helped to reflect on the emotional burden of this experience which had to some extent resulted from her identification with the patient and her family. In the group discussion her compassion was validated. She felt elated when she heard that many doctors can feel inadequate because they do not feel compassionate or empathetic enough towards their patients. She now realised that she was well endowed in this area and that she should not feel burdened, but rather privileged to have been put in that position. This opportunity to discuss and reflect on her feelings in this unfamiliar situation helped the student to become more aware of the problems of the threat to her professional boundaries in this non-clinical setting. While it helped her to appreciate her capacity for empathy, it also showed her how her empathic skills could be compromised by a lack of professional boundaries.

Handling embarrassment

A female student reported a 'situation' that occurred when she was observing the consultant running the genito-urinary oncology clinic. A consultant wanted to examine the perineal area of a frail 60-year-old man who had received radiotherapy for cancer of the prostate. The patient, without being asked for his consent to have the student present, shuffled to the examination couch and undressed himself from the waist down. He lay with his face towards the wall and his back towards the student and the consultant seemed unperturbed by his revealing position. He examined the perineal area and then suddenly stood up and swept out of the room, without giving an explanation, leaving the student standing behind this patient whose backside was fully exposed. The student had no idea where the consultant had gone and thought that he would be back in a few minutes. She found it difficult to know how to react. She did not know whether the examination had finished and whether to tell the patient to get dressed. She was totally unprepared for such an experience and was torn between the desire to get out of the consulting room and give him privacy and not wanting to leave him alone without an explanation. Finally, as a compromise, she positioned herself within the curtained enclosure in a way that allowed her not to be so close to him and look away.

Eventually the doctor returned with his trainee surgeon who had been involved in the patient's care. The doctor gave no explanation and made no apologies on his return. After the trainee had examined the area, the patient dressed and the consultation was brought to a close. The patient showed no sign of being displeased with the way his examination had been managed and left the consultation on amicable terms with everyone.

In the ensuing discussion the group sympathised with the student about the awkward nature of the situation and discussed ways of handling it. One of the leaders suggested that the intense awkwardness might have been alleviated by naming the feeling to herself and acknowledging the embarrassing nature of the situation to the patient. One of the students said that perhaps covering the patient with a blanket might have provided some relief. Another student said that the doctor seemed to be both unaware of the student's stage of professional development and her feelings. Another commented that it seemed as if a doctor who examined patients every day might become used to their nakedness and so was desensitised to embarrassment. The same leader emphasised that doctors are not expected to lose their sensitivity: he told the group about a medical exam candidate who was failed by the examiner because he said he had neglected to safeguard the privacy of a patient he was examining, by not drawing the curtains round his bed, on the grounds that the patient was blind!

The student felt that the discussion helped her identify the feelings involved and she felt more prepared to deal with similar situations in the future.

A disillusionment

A male student clerked a patient the day before she was due to have a hemi-colectomy for removal of a tumour of the bowel. She was friendly and willing to be clerked and let him take blood from her. He liked her for helping him and he explained the surgical procedure in detail to her and explored her anxieties about the cosmetic effect of the forthcoming colostomy.

The day after the operation he saw her again and realised now that there was something very wrong. She was in a side room and unresponsive: as the surgeons peeled the dressings to inspect the wound, he saw that the wound had dehisced and there was a gaping hole in the umbilical region close by the colostomy bag. He felt as if he was staring at an anatomical atlas: it was possible to see the layers of the abdominal wall, the skin, the fat and the muscle and through the wound, he could see her bowel! As soon as he saw the wound he felt a sense of revulsion that quickly turned into a morbid fascination. He felt that the lady had put her trust in medicine and in her surgeons and she had been badly let down. He felt that she had been put in the side room in order to hide this surgical failure. He felt guilty because he was a student of medicine and medicine had harmed her. He would feel embarrassed if he were to meet her again.

In our group discussion we reflected on the fact that medicine has a dark side and is not always ideal. Medical procedures sometimes fail for no good reason. The student hoped that if anything similar happened to him in the future, he would find the strength to admit the failure and offer an explanation to the patient.

Confusion of boundaries

A female medical student, whom I will call Kate, gave a very good account of confusion of boundaries in her example: she had just finished clerking a patient for her surgical presentation, when she was approached by another patient from the neighbouring bay. She was a slim, young woman dressed in casual clothes and roughly her age. She was friendly and in an excited way introduced herself as a final-year medical student from another medical school. She was complimentary about Kate's clerking, which she had overheard, and said that her own medical condition provided a really good history and she would be willing to offer herself to Kate for clerking.

She also gave Kate her mobile number so that she could be located at any time during her stay in hospital. Kate felt dazed by the experience.

She had just finished speaking to one patient and was not prepared for another encounter. When she met her again, a few hours later, this patient was again very chatty and started comparing her own medical school with Kate's: she gave her advice about textbooks and wanted to find out what Kate had been learning in lectures and spoke about her own frustrations as a medical student. However, when she started turning the pages of the medical records that Kate was carrying, our student closed the file as discreetly as she could and the student patient apologised.

In the group Kate talked of her feelings of uncertainty and disorientation in her role when confronted with a person who was at the same time patient, student and peer. The discussion helped her realise that this confusion of roles might be related to an over identification with someone of a similar age, who was also studying the same thing as she was. She could see that this confusion of boundaries might interfere with her clinical judgement and that this might be one of the reasons why the GMC discourages doctors from treating family members or friends.

Conclusion

A lot of emphasis is placed on the need for students to be empathic when they are in the presence of seriously ill patients. There is no doubt that without empathic attunement to their patients' emotional state there can be no true understanding of patients. However, such empathy can become a burden when a doctor is confronted again and again with the intense distress of his or her patients. It can threaten his personal boundaries and make him fall back on a frozen but calm state of emotional detachment. Learning about empathy in an environment that helps develop reflective self-awareness can help a medical student to learn to filter affective resonance over carefully graduated levels of connectedness and this may provide an antidote to the defence of detachment. Discussions in Balint groups represent a form of empathy exercise that can promote learning about empathic understanding, while respecting the developing students' professional identity.

The usefulness of this approach becomes obvious in the discussions students have in the Balint groups about their relationship to their cancer patients. While the first-clinical-year medical students are encouraged to get to know cancer patients as part of their oncology education, there is clearly a need for a space to consider the developing relationships that occur between these young and idealistic medical students and the vulnerable individuals who are experiencing such a life-threatening illness.

One female medical student presented a girl roughly her own age, who was suffering from cancer. She was single, lonely and obviously found the relationship with this student solacing and enjoyed their conversations but gradually she had become more demanding: she now wanted her to accompany her to all her medical appointments and she felt guilty at the thought of introducing limits on their relationship. She even invited her to go to a film with her but her mother fortunately thought that this would be rather inappropriate. Her assignment was coming to an end and she felt badly about stopping seeing her. She felt she ought to continue seeing her until her death. In the Balint group she had the opportunity to discuss this relationship and was encouraged to consider protecting her personal boundaries as an acceptable aspect of her developing professional identity.

Chapter 7

Students' experiences
of being in a Balint group

Noah Moran, Lara Curran and Paul Sackin

REFLECTIONS ON THE DEATH OF A YOUNG MAN

Noah Moran

Medical training seems to revel in pushing students into the clinical deep end. The burden of acquiring medical knowledge, coupled with achieving clinical competence, leaves little room for personal reflection and, at times, even less for the patient. My Balint group provided a venue where these shortcomings in my training could be overcome, but more than this it enabled me to gain an insight into the bigger picture and, as a consequence, change my approach to patients and their families.

Joining my Balint group shortly after finishing my surgical attachment, I was still immersed in a world of the acute abdomen where surgical acumen out-ranks bedside manner and all the stereotypes from years of watching medical dramas were confirmed. To my amazement, I loved it. I enjoyed the cama-raderie and felt my induction into the medical tribe complete as I followed my consultant in matching scrubs, listening to him regale the functions of his new mobile phone. Three years of pre-clinical training hadn't prepared me for life on the wards. My nervousness and anxiety found a hiding place within this surgical world; attending theatre most days allowed me to avoid the ward. Alongside the bonus of not running into the formidable ward sister, whose hatred for medical students was notorious, this strategy allowed me to avoid the patients. I knew each of my consultant's patients, not by name but by case; I had scrubbed in on many of their operations. Before long I was fully indoc-trinated into the surgical world, and with this came bravado, shortly followed by my ever-increasing ego, which swelled with each operation I assisted with. I was diligent: I took time to read notes and watch everything from induction of anaesthesia to the patient's return to the recovery suite. I would clerk patients mostly just before their procedure. Minutes before they were due to be walked around to the anaesthetic room, I was there detailing presenting complaints, listing differentials and ensuring that in the quiet time before an operation I was there asking questions.

Joining my Balint group, I did not know what to expect. The introductory talk had covered the logistics and basic concepts, but I still had little idea what it was about. In truth I had opted to enrol in a Balint group to avoid writing a reflective essay[1] (this was a curriculum alternative). I resented my feelings being subjectively assessed and arbitrarily given a grade. I was a good talker, so the opportunity of having a captive audience to listen to me was not one I was going to pass up. Most meetings would begin in the same way. As people arrived, we would exchange stories of various firms and placements, chatting happily away until we were invited to begin by one of the leaders who would invite someone to share an experience of being with a patient with the group. A silence would fall across the group as our eyes fell to the floor avoiding eye contact, until someone would break the silence and say: 'I have a patient'. We shared a common nervousness; this environment was totally alien to us. Although we had been together for 3 years, it was commonplace to turn up to a tutorial and meet people for the first time, which was not surprising given our year had 400 students.

As someone shared their story we would listen and learn about a troublesome patient or situation. The presenting student was given time before we would explore further the elements of the story that had struck a chord with us or which we felt needed clarification. After this, the person who presented would step back while the rest of the group discussed the patient, before moving on to another case. This was the first time I had heard a case presentation without thinking about a surgical sieve to determine a differential diagnosis. As people explained their case, they painted a picture of the patient: we all added to this image with questions, as we hypothesised about the patient's agenda and motivations. This patient-centered approach was new to me and I revelled in exploring the patient's perspective, without having to consider their medical story.

I found myself revisiting patients I had met during my surgical attachment. One patient repeatedly returned to my mind. James was a 32-year-old medically well man except that his weight in stones matched his age. He was admitted for an elective gastric bypass. The hospital I was attached to had invested heavily (pardon the pun) in new bariatric facilities, so as to offer weight-loss surgery. Obesity, despite affecting one in four people, is still a source of great stigma, making it an easy target for hospital gallows humour. James underwent his surgery without complication. I was on intensive care when he woke from his anaesthetic. James's bulky frame filled the extra-large, reinforced bed specially purchased to accommodate bariatric patients. I visited him most days on one ward round or another. I had spoken to him briefly before his operation and I remember thinking that his history was boring: 'A 32-year-old failed dieter, father of two, presents for gastric bypass with banding; medically stable with Type 2 diabetes and hypertension, and no previous surgery.' James struggled to leave intensive care. Post operatively, he developed a pulmonary embolus and later a chest infection. When he did find his way to the surgical ward, he managed to pick up an MRSA infection, giving his wound very little chance to heal, and eventually he developed cellulitis. This latest infection brought him back to intensive care, where he stayed for the next 3 weeks. His 5-day post operative stay turned into 5 weeks. James became a regular fixture on the ward round. At times I would see him two or three times a day punching in texts onto his mobile phone. You could hear the vibration tone of the phone against his bedside table across the ward when he received messages. When he died over the weekend just before Christmas, I wasn't there. I found out about his death the following Monday.

I found myself going over his history again and again. How old were his children? Why had I not seen them at some point during his prolonged stay? Why did he never complain? Everything that could have gone wrong did and yet he never complained. I could not get the image of him texting out of my mind: who was he texting? Alongside these questions, I found myself feeling profoundly guilty about making jokes about him. At one point he had needed a CT scan and he would not fit in the hospital's scanner. When I learned that the zoo had been contacted to utilise their extra-large machine, I made sure that I passed on this story to my fellow students.

I brought James's case to a Balint session. As I told his story I realised how little I knew about him and I felt ashamed when I explained the jokes I had made about his size. Discussing his case, the group demonstrated a concern for him that I had failed to show when he was alive. They asked about his motivation to undergo surgery. Thinking about it, I realised that he had struggled with obesity all his life and that this operation must have represented hope for him. Sharing my feelings about James, I recognised that having struggled with my own weight, I could have used this shared relationship to facilitate a better relationship. Instead I used the common values of the other members of the surgical team to make jokes. This experience, alongside others from my Balint group, has shaped my future patient interactions. I recognised that, as a student, I benefited from the luxury of time. I could explore non-clinical areas with patients, while at the same time formulating a good differential diagnosis. The benefit of this approach was that I could now form a better relationship with the patient: it would be a relationship based on a mutual dialogue, where we both shared experiences and found common values.

My patient histories are now unrecognisable compared with those from my first surgical firm, not only because of my clinical training, but because of the insight I have gained through completing a Balint group. Discussing the alternative agenda of a consultation has opened up a world beyond the findings on physical examination and the differential diagnosis. I have learnt to think more about my patient as a person rather than as a presentation or a disease. My interactions with patients now follow a far less regimented approach. Whilst obtaining 'the history of the presenting complaint', I now have the confidence to explore less traditional medical subjects: exploring my patient's ideas and concerns, I try to avoid overly structured models from medical school teaching and opt for my own strategies in which my initial approach is aimed at establishing a relationship affirming trust. I am not just trying to build a rapport with the patient, but trying to do more: focusing on contextual questions rather than asking, 'How bad is the pain on a scale of one to ten?', I ask 'How does this impact on your daily life? What does this pain stop you from doing?' This technique allows for greater insights into the patient's perspectives. My experience of the Balint group has taught me to appreciate the patient's agenda during a consultation. Taking time to find out what is important to the patient reveals that their perspective may not tally with my own views and acknowledging and exploring these differences allows for better trust and mutual respect to develop, which permits a better exchange of information and knowledge.

Reflecting on my experience within the Balint group, I am grateful for this opportunity to share with and learn from others. I have not only gained an insight into my patients and those of my colleagues, but also an appreciation of the patient's agenda that has changed my approach to patients. For me, involvement in this group gave me space to reflect, to appreciate the subtleties of consultations and to apply these lessons to clinical practice.

WHAT IS THE ROLE OF A MEDICAL STUDENT IN THE CARE OF PATIENTS?

Lara Curran

During the time I spent in the Balint group, I found that one particular unifying theme ran through the sessions, which was a frequently recurring topic of discussion. This was the group's struggle with the limits and constraints of the medical student–patient relationship. This issue arose in case discussions, varying from the interaction with a patient who expressed suicidal thoughts, to the relationships forged with the patients struggling with cancer. Being clinical medical students enables us for the first time to take an extensive, and often what feels like an invasive, look into a patient's illness. This privilege can sometimes feel undeserved, as we often have little or no capacity to improve the patient's medical condition. At times I found it easy to feel as if I were taking something from the patient, whether it was their time or personal information, without being able to give anything useful back. It is tempting to feel that the interaction has been more for my benefit than for the patient's, almost exploiting their illness for its educational value. This ethos seemed to contradict the patient-centred approach that has been instilled in us from the beginning of medical school. It left many of us unsure as to how our 'role' in hospital should be defined and how far we could extend its boundaries to improve the care of patients. In the most extreme cases, might our interactions with patients have caused them emotional distress that was counterproductive to their recovery?

My prior knowledge of Balint groups was restricted to a 150-word synopsis, provided to all students in our year, to help us select an SSC module for the forthcoming year. Although the idea of a course that seemed removed from the traditional 'scientific' SSC modules typically on offer was appealing, I had few expectations of what this type of discussion would entail and no idea of the impact the course would have on my thinking about my interactions with patients.

As I think back to our first session, I remember a feeling of awkwardness that hung in the small room in the Psychotherapy Department, where we would meet for an hour[2] each Monday evening. Until this point in our medical education, we had often been asked how or why we were expected to do something, but never how we felt about doing it. In a room full of medical students, never shy to offer up answers, we nervously sat in silence waiting for one of us to pluck up the courage to speak. One of my lasting memories is of how comfortable our group facilitators seemed to be as they allowed us to sit without saying a word. However uneasy we felt, they appeared relaxed, as though our very reluctance to speak about our experiences spoke volumes.

As the weeks went on, we became more comfortable as a group and accustomed to the format of the discussions. One member would put forward a story without interruption and then allow the others to discuss the issues that had arisen from it. I was amazed that entire patient narratives could be retold without the mention of investigations or test results or the typical jargon that litters medical history taking. Where previously stories recounted to us had been ones of illness, suddenly they became stories of people: as a result they began to have a whole new and fascinating dimension. It was so much more engaging to hear about the impact that these events had had on the people involved, as too often before I had wondered why these details were neglected or even omitted in the clinical histories I had heard on the ward.

I enjoyed listening to the stories of the other students and often took comfort from the realisation that I wasn't alone in feeling overwhelmed by the sudden exposure to a vast range of human emotions I was witnessing on the wards. I saw the Balint group as a welcome and, at times, almost necessary outlet for some of the frustrations that had naturally built up during my first term as a clinical student. Despite this I was hesitant to put forward my own story to the rest of the group. It was only at the sixth session that I finally decided to share with the group my experience with a particular patient I had met earlier in the year. This was an encounter that seemed to highlight some of the complex issues that had been a recurrent theme of our discussions within the group.

For my first clinical attachment, I was assigned to the haematological malignancy ward to begin a 6-week placement in oncology. Although I was excited to begin clinical medicine, I was also extremely apprehensive, as this wasn't my first experience of hospital oncology. The previous Christmas I had been diagnosed with Hodgkin's lymphoma and had spent most of the previous year undergoing chemotherapy. Although I was lucky enough to make a full recovery, the experience and all the emotions that had accompanied it were still at the forefront of my mind, especially as my remission had only come a few months before term began. To my surprise, the time I spent on this oncology placement was not nearly as harrowing as I had expected. I found I was able to separate my own experiences from those of the very ill, and often elderly, patients I saw on ward rounds. Creating this wall between them and me, patient and medical student, was the way I was best able to cope. Listening to some of the discussions in Balint group, I wondered if this might be a tool, commonly used by medical professionals to maintain a degree of emotional detachment that might be protective.

The wall that I had built up was less easy to maintain when I came into contact with one particular patient. As part of my teaching, an oncology registrar had asked me to clerk a patient on the ward. I asked the staff nurse if she knew of any suitable patients who wouldn't mind speaking to me, and she helpfully directed me to one who was being treated in a side room. I was warned that this was a patient who was at risk of sepsis, caused by having too few of a certain type of white blood cells (neutropaenia) as a result of her myelosupressive chemotherapy regime: this meant I would have to wear a mask, gloves and a full protective apron. I was told that the patient was very friendly and would have no problem talking to me. She turned out to be a 33-year-old lady who had only recently been diagnosed with acute myeloid leukaemia. She had initially presented to hospital with an acute onset of shortness of breath and recurrently bleeding gums, having previously felt completely well.

On entering the room, I instantly felt uncomfortable and awkward, as I attempted to build up a reasonable rapport with the patient with a mask obscuring half my face. Despite this, she was extremely understanding and talkative, which began to make me feel more relaxed. I asked her if she would mind if I asked a few questions about how she had come to be in hospital and as the nurse predicted, she was very obliging. From talking to her I could gather that she was a well-educated woman in a high-pressured job in the financial sector and that she had three young children, all under the age of six. She was originally from abroad, but had been living in London for 5 years, where she had met her husband. Her diagnosis and the speed at which her life had been completely transformed had obviously come as a huge shock. The conversation began with some general questions about her life, which were well received. The discussion became more difficult as we moved away from these 'safe' topics to begin talking about the reasons for her medical admission. I discovered that she had completed the first cycle of her chemotherapy and was being considered for a bone marrow transplant. She had lost all her hair in the past few days and was starting to feel the full force of her intensive regimen.

As she recounted some of the side effects of her treatment, it became obvious that the mood of our conversation was beginning to change. It wasn't only the patient who was starting to feel uncomfortable; for me this was the first time

I had heard someone else talk at length about their experiences with cancer and I found it impossible not to draw parallels between our two stories. In particular I could empathise with the shock that she had felt at her diagnosis and her fear of losing her hair. She was obviously tired and had been nauseous throughout the night. She was in a strange medical ward, away from her family and friends and completely removed from the life she had known only a few weeks before. This was a patient at her most vulnerable and I had been sent to learn from her terrible experience. I tried to steer her away from discussing her treatment, but it was an area we found ourselves revisiting. I felt as though our conversation might provide her with an outlet to discuss her problems and express her frustration about the situation she had found herself in. During my own illness I had found that discussing my fears with those closest to me was often too difficult and it was the nurses with whom I had sometimes opened up the most.

At one point during our conversation, the patient mentioned the horrible nausea she could feel a few days after her treatment. As she talked candidly about her experience of chemotherapy, she gradually became more outwardly emotional: this was my first experience of seeing a distressed patient and I felt at a loss to think of something helpful to say. I couldn't help but be reminded of my own treatment and without thinking carefully enough, I said, 'I know, it must be horrible for you. I'm sorry.' At this point, the patient suddenly got angry at my response to her distress. She countered, 'What do you mean you know? You are so young and have no idea what I'm going through.'

This kind of conversation is an example of a situation that can arise unexpectedly and test the boundaries of the student–patient relationship. I felt that I had caused her distress and that my response had unintentionally belittled the ordeal she had been through. Both the patient and I had made assumptions; I imagined that by trying to empathise with her I might have been able to comfort her, while she had come to the completely reasonable conclusion that I was unlikely to know how terrible chemotherapy could make you feel. In a sense, I think this encounter exposed how patients can feel a wall that separates them from doctors. This wall means that both patients and doctors see themselves as being in completely separate groups, i.e. doctors see themselves as treating people who are ill, and they don't imagine themselves becoming ill and in need of treatment. From this perspective, it could be easy for a patient to make an assumption that a medical student has no experience of what they are going through. I think in this particular case, my age might also have created a barrier in our communication and the patient might have construed my response as being patronising, given that I was only 21.

In the instant that the patient challenged my response, I felt torn between maintaining a professional distance by keeping quiet, and the natural instinct to try to explain what I had meant by my comment. I could completely sympathise with the frustration that made her respond in this way. I think that part of the emotional isolation that can sometimes occur in such an evocative illness as cancer is the tendency for a patient to feel that other 'healthy' people have no idea of what they are going through. In a strange and frightening environment, faced with the daunting prospect of chemotherapy, I can't blame my patient at all for allowing her fear to express itself in this way.

I decided it would be better to try to put aside my preconceived idea of what the medical student–patient relationship should be, and attempt to relate to the patient at a more personal level. I explained that I was really sorry if what I had said had come across in the wrong way, but that I could understand some of what she was going through, as I had also been through chemotherapy. As soon as I said this, I was scared that I had crossed a boundary, yet it felt like the best way to deal with the situation. Interestingly, this confession transformed the dynamics of the conversation. The patient instantly switched from being defensive and seemed to adopt an almost apologetic tone. Above all, I noticed her surprise and how interested she was to find out about how well I had tolerated my treatment. Indeed, it might have given her some sort of comfort to see someone who had been in a similar situation and who had now recovered. I felt for the first time in the conversation that I was able to provide her with some real reassurance about her treatment.

As I finished retelling my story to the Balint group, I remember feeling some of the anxieties of that day return. In contrast to some of the other stories we had heard in the group, this discussion focused on my reaction as much as it did the patient's. I had been reticent to share my experience with the group, as I worried that they might disagree with my actions, confirming my worst fears that I had overstepped a professional boundary. A more terrifying prospect perhaps was that the story had exposed so much about my own personal experiences, as previously only one other member of the group had been aware that I had just recovered from a cancer.

During the course of our meetings, the topic of cancer had come up on many occasions. It seemed as though every session was linked to this illness in some way. Each time I struggled with whether it would be appropriate to tell the rest of the group about my own experience. In one sense I felt I had now gained a different perspective on what it felt like to be both a patient and part of a health care team, something that could have been a useful contribution to this discussion. On the other hand, I felt concerned that by talking about it I might make the other members of the group feel less free to discuss the topic in front of me. Up till my presentation, our discussion of cancer had been extensive; while I found most of it very interesting, some of the more frank retellings of patients' struggles with terminal illness were a little harder to hear: these were stories that most would not have shared in the presence of someone who had just had cancer themselves.

In this context, I was very apprehensive about how the group would react. Yet everyone was supportive and understanding of the difficulties the meeting with my patient had uncovered. We agreed that the patient might have found some comfort in being able to speak to someone who had been in a similar position. I had felt lucky that the conversation with my patient had ended so positively. We had finished our conversation on excellent terms and all the frustrations that we had both experienced seemed dispelled.

Despite this, for some time after my meeting with this patient, I continued to worry that I had made the wrong decision by discussing my own health with her. I posed this question to our Balint group. After much debate we came to the view, as so often occurs in medicine, that there could be no simple answer. Every decision, whether it is a clinical one or an emotional one, is patient and context specific. Much as in the way that we are taught to spot the subtlest clinical sign that may guide management, care must be taken to look for those emotional cues that inform how we interact with our patients. The approach we choose to take with one patient may be entirely inappropriate in another context, and each interaction must be judged carefully. Since then I have seen many cancer patients but never again have I felt the urge to talk about my illness with them. I think that this one case was unique in that the patient challenged me directly and I had felt instinctively that in that moment my subsequent explanation to her had been the right thing to do.

Although this was uncomfortable at the time, the experience has taught me an invaluable lesson. It has given me an insight into how patients view medical students and how sensitive we must be to their emotional fragility when they are so ill. It also showed me that the most effective communication comes when we treat them as people, not just as patients. While maintaining professional boundaries is clearly integral to medicine, being able to relate to patients as people is of paramount importance in creating a good relationship. I have also begun to realise that I underestimated the impact that my conversations with patients had on their care. I hope that in the case of my patient, allowing her to vent her frustrations and attempting to comfort her by breaking down the wall I had built between us may have helped her in some way.

On reflection, I think that the role that we have as medical students is constantly changing. With every patient and every new experience I have, I feel that my idea of what it means to be a medical student is evolving. With every new interaction a whole new set of challenges arises and having a forum like a Balint group to share our thoughts together as a medical community is a vital part of our continuing development as thoughtful clinicians.

MY EXPERIENCE OF BEING IN A STUDENT GROUP RUN BY MICHAEL BALINT

Paul Sackin

In October 1966 I had completed my pre-clinical studies and done an intercalated pharmacology BSc. I had enjoyed the pharmacology but felt that it was not an area I wished to pursue as a career. The course had also made me more aware of my limitations in the technical aspects of laboratory work. My unsuccessful attempts to catch the appropriate laboratory mouse from those in the cage had dubbed me as 'not one of our best handlers'. I thought that a career that dealt primarily with people rather than technical matters might be better for me.

My clinical training at University College Hospital (UCH) started with an introductory course and then I was attached to a medical firm. We had plenty of time to talk to patients who had a whole variety of diseases, often very serious. It was challenging, but also rewarding, to try and answer patients' questions, particularly about their prognosis, that they were too frightened to ask a more senior member of the firm. To help with this work we had regular tutorials with a psychiatric trainee who was 'attached' to the firm. I found these enormously useful. I was therefore most excited when it was announced that seminars led by Michael Balint would start for our year in early 1967. Attendance was voluntary. I had, of course, never heard of Balint but the seminars were promoted by two of the psychiatry consultants, Roger Tredgold and Heinz Wolff, whose lectures on our introductory course had very much impressed me. As I remember it, Tredgold and Wolff explained that the seminars would help us to understand our patients better. This might be a bit uncomfortable but it would pay off in terms of working with the patients.

However, I had a dilemma. The Balint seminars were to be held weekly at 5pm, on exactly the same day as chorus rehearsals for the University College Opera. I had been in two previous opera productions and had enjoyed them enormously. I had been in rehearsals for Donizetti's Poliuto since October 1966 and I was reluctant to drop out before the performances in March 1967. What should I do? After much thought I decided to stick with the opera. I reasoned that this would be my last chance to take part in such a production, whereas the Balint work was ongoing and to miss the first 2 months of seminars was a small sacrifice in the longer term. It could well be that this decision was the most crucial one in shaping my future career. The Balint seminars had been so well 'sold' to our year that around 20 students turned up. This was too many for this group and many of my fellow students were disappointed and left it. By the time I joined in March 1967 the group had settled to around 12 regular members. Had I joined in January I could well have been put off Balint's approach for ever.

First impressions

I went along to my first group wondering what to expect. Balint seemed a benign enough man. In 1967 he would have been 71 years old and I guess he looked that sort of age. He had very thick glasses and could read only with difficulty. Mary Hare, a consultant psychotherapist, co-led, though as I remember it she made few contributions unless Balint was away, when she led the group on her own. However, she was busy writing down everything that was said in the group, I believe verbatim. I did not realise it at the time, but Balint's groups had always been for 'research cum training' (in that order) and the student group was no exception.

Balint always started with 'who has a case?' My memory is that in the 90 minutes that we had, two new cases and often two follow-up cases were discussed. As I recall it there only seemed to be one 'rule' – case notes were not permitted. This struck me as strange – but not for long. It soon became clear that what the presenter recalled, or didn't recall, was much more significant than what was written down. My most vivid memory of these early seminars was that Balint's approach was what we now call 'evidence based'. He kept asking us to speculate about what might be going on, based on what we had heard (or hadn't heard). So, for example, if we didn't hear whether a middle-aged patient was married or not, we were encouraged to consider whether there might be some problem in this area of the patient's life. Often the 'speculations' seemed quite wild but very often, when we heard a follow-up report, they were absolutely right. Most of us rapidly developed a love-hate relationship with Balint. His speculations (or rather encouraging the group members to make them) always seemed to be right – how maddening! As a very naive 21-year-old my eyes were opened to the extraordinary lives that so many people led and to the difficulties many patients put up with. I felt I was learning a huge amount about people but I said very little in the group and did not present a patient for some time.

Aberdeen

Not long after I had started in the group, Balint received an invitation to lecture about the student groups to the department of psychiatry in Aberdeen. He replied that he couldn't possibly give the flavour of the groups in a lecture; the only way was a demonstration. To his, and our, surprise, the Aberdonians readily agreed to this. So, Balint and about a dozen members of the combined junior and senior student groups boarded a night sleeper train for Aberdeen one Friday evening. Balint generously plied us with whiskey on the journey.

We ran groups for most of Saturday and Sunday but also had some free time to be shown round the city. We were tastefully accommodated for Saturday night in the ECT ward of the local psychiatric hospital. As I remember it, the groups ran much as they did back home but there was time after each session for the audience to join in a discussion of what had gone on – very much like the 'fishbowl' sessions that are almost de rigueur at modern Balint conferences. The Aberdonians appeared to find the groups very interesting and there was much discussion both during the sessions and informally afterwards. To this day I still feel somewhat guilty that I did not say a word in the group during the entire weekend. I was still quite diffident in the group back home but in Aberdeen the presence of senior students (a year or 18 months ahead of me) was really inhibiting. They seemed so confident in their contributions.

My first case

After a couple of months or so in the group I finally plucked up courage to present a case. I had been quite stunned when a 50-year-old patient asked me when it would be safe to resume sexual intercourse, after the myocardial infarction that he had suffered from. I had, of course, no idea of the answer to this question and was extremely embarrassed to be asked it. I think I felt a touch of anger with the patient that he had 'landed' me with this question – until I realised that the house officer (now called Foundation Year doctor) was female and the trainee physician and his consultant were not very accessible. Maybe the Balint group could help – but was it really OK to present the case as I didn't really know anything about the man?

In those days a heart attack was treated with ten days' bed rest and I would go and see the patient each day. He didn't have much to say and all I remembered was that he was married and had a 10-year-old son. As the discussion went on, and Balint encouraged the group to speculate, I realised that I knew rather more than I had thought about this man. For example, he had said that he worked abroad a lot. He had married late and was 40 when his son was born. Might he be trying to please women other than his wife? Could intercourse be more important to him than at first seemed to be the case? I was left with a lot of questions and a much heightened curiosity about him. In addition Balint – true to his scientific background – asked the group if anyone knew the answer to my patient's question. Nobody did, so we were asked to look up the literature on intercourse after a heart attack and bring our findings to a future seminar. In the end I told this man he could resume intercourse 6 weeks after his heart attack. It's a pity that detractors of Balint and his method were not aware of his evidence-based approach.

Progress in the groups

The real value of the groups for me was during my junior student attachments to the medical and surgical wards. As patients were in hospital generally for far longer than they are nowadays, it was possible to spend time with them and test out the suggestions from the group. I remember how the most outlandish speculations made in the group so often turned out to be right. I also became aware of how sad some people's lives were and that easy solutions were not forthcoming. I have never quite forgotten a middle-aged woman patient presented by a fellow student who in childhood had been 'so delicate she had to go upstairs backwards'. This label seemed to stick with her and the impression we got in the group was that she had had a miserable life, as she couldn't and maybe later wouldn't, do anything useful or gratifying.

For some reason my year was the last year in which separate junior and senior groups were run. This seemed to be because the number of participants in my year had dwindled and few new students from the year below me wished to join. I was never clear why this was. For a while the seminars continued reasonably successfully as one group but numbers continued to fall. By this time my colleagues and I were in our second clinical year and spent time in shorter attachments. This meant that we did not usually have 'our own' patients and had limited continuity. Furthermore, some of our attachments were away from University College Hospital (UCH), even out of London on occasions. Thus, attendance was difficult, we rarely had cases to present and several more students left. After a while, the three or four of us in my year who continued to attend reasonably regularly were to some extent coming in order to keep the group viable. We had quite a lot of discussion in the group as to why the numbers were so small, but it was difficult to draw any clear conclusions. During this time one of the students in the year below me, who had been a group member, committed suicide. This tragedy led to a huge amount of heart searching in the group – had we ignored our colleague's calls for help? – and almost certainly hastened the demise of the group. I can't remember exactly when the group ended but I suspect it was when my colleagues and I went on our electives, in spring 1969.

The groups in context

I remember that in the discussions about the falling membership of the group, Balint appeared almost paranoid about the consultants at UCH. He felt that they were completely against his approach and would not offer any support in encouraging students to join the group. To some extent this was probably true – it was hard to see many of the surgeons, for example, rushing to support the groups. But I still remember two physicians – and there were probably others – who deeply impressed me with their holistic approach to patients. One was David Edwards who had a special interest in grossly overweight patients. He acted as a mentor to me during my work with one of these patients, whom I followed up well beyond the time I was attached to Dr Edwards' firm. Eventually he urged me to wean myself away from the patient, a wise thing to do. The other memorable consultant was Simon Yudkin, a paediatrician. His outpatient clinics were the highlight of our week during our paediatric attachment and attendance was almost always 100%. Despite 14 students and at least one nurse in the room, Yudkin somehow managed to form an intense relationship with the child and his/her family – we could see the family dynamics playing out in front of us. My memory of Yudkin was made much more poignant as he died suddenly over the Easter break of my paediatric attachment.

These consultants showed me just how patients could, and should, be treated and how the Balint group might help me achieve such a goal. However, it was not until I spent 2 weeks with Philip Hopkins, as my 'voluntary' general practice attachment, that I realised the full value of the Balint approach to patients. Hopkins was in the group that led to the classic book, *The Doctor, his*

Patient and the Illness (Balint, 1964) and was the founder of the Balint Society. Without these key attachments I wonder if I would have realised the full value of the student Balint group or of the satisfaction of a career in general practice, trying to live up to the standards of my enlightened predecessors. I hope this account of the Balint group, attended about 45 years ago, shows how the combination of the group experience and having role models practising in a holistic way are key to successful education in patient-centred medicine.

Notes

1 Initially the Balint group students were exempt from a general requirement for first year clinical students to write a reflective essay. Since this student attended his Balint group, writing a reflective essay has also become a requirement of attending a student Balint group.
2 At this time the student Balint groups only lasted for 1 hour per session.

Chapter 8

Research into the two schemes

Jessica Yakeley

Patient-centred medicine

The Student Psychotherapy Scheme and Balint groups are teaching methods about the role of emotions in illness and the doctor–patient relationship that are grounded in patient-centred medicine. The term 'patient-centred medicine'[1] was first introduced in the medical literature by Balint in a paper describing his teaching seminars during the 1960s for medical students at University College Hospital with the object of studying emotional problems of patients admitted to the wards (Balint et al., 1969). Balint was attempting to create a different approach to the medical treatment of patients from what he felt was the prevalent attitude at that time, which he called 'illness-centred medicine'. The illness-centred approach, which was based on observations from an uninvolved 'objective' observer, was concerned with body parts or discrete illnesses, and encouraged an impersonal relationship with the patient where the doctor relied on tests such as X-rays, external reports and laboratory examinations to inform diagnosis and treatment without the patient's involvement. By contrast, patient-centred medicine required a participating or involved observer, who thought in terms of personality difficulties and disturbed human relationships, and a relationship with the patient where information was shared. Balint highlighted how emotional problems in patients occupied a 'kind of no-man's land: they are the province of neither the physician nor the psychiatrist' (Balint et al., 1969, p. 249). For Balint, patient-centred medicine involved the explicit study of emotions and elucidating the link between the patient's physical symptoms and emotional disturbance.

There is now a large body of research demonstrating that effective clinical communication is linked with a number of significant positive outcomes, including patient satisfaction, recall, adherence and concordance with treatment, well-being, physical and psychological outcome, and patient safety (Shapiro et al., 2009). Moreover, there is evidence that the majority of complaints and lawsuits against doctors cite poor communication as the main cause of the patient's grievance (Tamblyn et al., 2007). These findings have led to the assessment and teaching of communication skills becoming central components of undergraduate medical education in the UK (von Fragstein et al., 2008). 'Patient-centredness' as a theoretical approach has become widely accepted as an essential feature underpinning high-quality patient care and now forms a central part of undergraduate medical communication curricula. Respectful partnerships with patients, patient autonomy, patient choice and self-determined needs are all emphasised as being key aspects of the patient-centred approach that should be at the core of health care interactions and the doctor–patient relationship. Students are taught that respect for others and a commitment to equality and diversity are at the centre of all effective clinical communication (von Fragstein et al., 2008).

The place of emotions

However, the place of emotions within medical training and practice remains elusive. Emotional issues that may arise in both doctor and patient are often still relegated to Balint's 'no-mans land' where they remain unspoken and unexamined. Although 'handling emotions' is listed as one of the specific issues to be taught in the UK consensus statement on the content of communication curricula in undergraduate medical education (von Fragstein et al., 2008), the emphasis is on teaching behavioural skills such as eye contact, attentive listening, balance of open and closed questions, summarising, signposting and 'chunking information'. Within North American medical education, it has been observed that an explicit commitment to traditional professional values of empathy, compassion and altruism conceals a tacit commitment to behaviours grounded in ethics of detachment, self-interest and objectivity, promoting a culture of emotional detachment and distancing from patients (Coulehan and Williams, 2001). This may result in wide-scale 'professional alexithymia' in which emotions within the doctor–patient relationship cannot be recognised, processed or regulated (Shapiro, 2011). Exposed to the role models of their physician teachers, medical students may interpret 'handling emotions' as meaning distancing oneself from emotional contact. They pick up cognitive or behavioural strategies to respond to displays of emotions in the patient, such as offering minimal empathy and not enquiring further into the patient's source of distress, or engaging in 'blocking behaviours' such as changing the subject, breaking eye contact or ignoring the patient's tears. Students also learn to view their own emotions with suspicion: positive emotions, such as liking or feeling attracted to patients, are viewed as potentially interfering with the doctor's ability to make objective professional judgements about diagnosis and treatment, and at worse may lead to boundary violations. Acknowledging that one may have negative emotions about a patient, such as feeling irritated, angry, contemptuous or hateful, may make the student feel that they are violating the respect that they are meant to show to the patient and so lead the student to deny their emotional responses completely.

Empathy has been identified as a key component of professionalism, and one of the goals in all medical education curricula in both North America and the UK is the development of empathy in learners. Thus, the Royal College of Psychiatrists' core curriculum defines three principle aims for the undergraduate medical course specific to clinical psychiatry teaching: (a) to provide students with knowledge of the main psychiatric disorders, the principles underlying modern psychiatric theory, commonly used treatments and a basis on which to develop this knowledge; (b) to assist students to develop the necessary skills to apply this knowledge in clinical situations; and (c) to encourage students to develop appropriate attitudes necessary to respond empathically to psychological distress in all medical settings (Cooper et al., 2011, p. 31). Shapiro (2011), however, draws attention to the fate of the empathy construct in medical education research and the curriculum with a shift towards defining empathy as a purely cognitive process. Empathy is identified as an objective, rational, accurate, intellectual and ultimately positive process, to be distinguished from sympathy, which is regarded as emotional, self-indulgent and potentially dangerous (leading, for example, to burnout or boundary breaking). Students are taught empathy via a set of cognitive and behavioural skills at the expense of facilitating emotional awareness and reflection. Students learn that emotions are to be avoided or denied, instead of being explicitly taught how to recognise, calibrate and act upon their affective responses appropriately and proportionately to clinical circumstances.

Why research is important

Research is a method of investigation or experimentation that involves the collection and analysis of data, information or facts for the advancement of human knowledge. It involves a process of determining specific research questions or hypotheses so that theories may be tested and revised. Conducting research is necessary in order to accumulate sufficient evidence to support one's ideas and theories, to convince others of their validity, and to ensure their dissemination and survival. In his paper on training medical students in patient-centred medicine, Balint himself appeared cognisant of the importance of researching his approach, in listing the particular issues, or research questions, that he wished to study:'(1) Could this approach lead to a better understanding of the illness? (2) What kind of help could a student be expected to give his or her patient when adopting this approach? (3) What demands could we make on the student and he or she on himself or herself? (4) What kind of training could be offered to the student to help his or her patients in this different way?' (Balint, 1969, p. 250).

If we wish to convince others of the significance of the role of emotions and emotional communication within medical training and practice, we need to follow Balint in harnessing our enthusiasm and curiosity into formulating research questions and establishing processes of systematic inquiry to test our theoretical frameworks and to demonstrate the benefits of our specific teaching methods. In doing so, we may draw on the growing body of research that has accumulated since Balint's introduction of the patient-centred approach that demonstrates that patients' emotions may have a significant impact on clinical outcomes. For example, sadness and anger may amplify the experience of pain, depression may interfere with compliance to diabetic regimens, and mood states, independent from compliance, have been shown to influence outcomes in medical conditions such as diabetes, myocardial infarction and cancer (Shapiro, 2011). Moreover, many studies have shown that emotions influence the behaviour of both patients and physicians in decision making, information processing and interpersonal attitudes in the doctor–patient relationship (Oatley et al., 2006; Isen et al., 1991; Shapiro, 2011). There is also evidence that acknowledging a patient's emotional distress is essential for effective discussion of clinical issues with the patient and associated with increased compliance and positive outcome (Smith et al., 2011).

Since the inception of the UCL Student Psychotherapy Scheme and the establishment of related schemes in other countries there have been various attempts to conduct systematic research into the impact and outcomes of this teaching method. Similarly, both qualitative and quantitative research studies have been undertaken to investigate the nature and impact of Balint groups as a method of learning about the doctor–patient relationship for medical students at our own medical school and at medical schools in other countries. Before describing and critiquing these studies in further detail, it is helpful to reflect on what such research is trying to achieve, and to be aware of the many difficulties and ambiguities inherent in attempting to investigate the field of emotional and interpersonal communications in which any degree of objectivity is hard to establish.

For example, one approach might be to define the aims of the specific teaching method and to conduct a study investigating whether the teaching course achieves those aims. For the Student Psychotherapy Scheme, one of its main objectives is to enable students to become more aware of the role of emotions within the doctor–patient relationship. But how do we measure emotional communication or an individual's awareness of their own or another person's feelings? As noted above, empathy has been identified as a key construct in this area, but the focus has been on its cognitive and behavioural aspects, which are easier to define and observe than any emotional component. Emotions fluctuate according to circumstance and context, they may be difficult to name or differentiate, and acknowledging them to oneself, let alone others, may be influenced by many factors including peer pressure, fear of disapproval or exposure, or cultural issues, to name but a few. In other words, the data that we are attempting to collect – in this case, an ability in the student or doctor to reflect upon both their own and their patients' emotional states and to use these in the best interests of the patient's care – eludes precise, consistent and reliable measurement.

We should rightly be interested in quantitative or outcome research that investigates the effects of the teaching on the student, for example, whether participation in a Balint group increases students' knowledge of the doctor–patient relationship. We should also be interested in investigating unintended or unexpected outcomes of our teaching methods, for example, the influence of participation in a Student Psychotherapy Scheme on career choice. We need to be mindful of how the aims of our teaching intersect with the wider aims of undergraduate medical education, such as enabling the student to deliver safer patient care. Improving understanding of clinical risk and patient safety are not only long-term goals of learning but are also live issues for the student participating in the Student Psychotherapy Scheme in which he or she becomes the primary therapist with responsibility for delivering treatment for a real, not simulated, patient. In other words, this particular teaching method has direct effects on clinical outcomes for patients that need to be considered, as well as on learning outcomes for the student.

Moreover, we should be interested in the nature and methods by which any demonstrated outcomes of our teaching have been achieved. For example, if we demonstrate that students who have completed the Student Psychotherapy Scheme have an increased understanding of concepts such as transference and countertransference, is this a result of the supervisor's teaching or recommended reading, discussion with peers within the supervision group, the live experience of becoming a transference object for their patient and experience of countertransference feelings, or due to factors that have nothing to do with the scheme, such as attending a lecture on psychotherapy that is available to all medical students or due to specific personality traits of the individual student? Elucidating some of these different factors will depend upon the design of the research study – whether the study involves randomisation to a control group, or whether it uses qualitative methods of investigation, such as asking a sample of participating students about their experience of the teaching and analysing their responses with a grounded theory approach.

Finally, we should be interested in the type of knowledge that the student learns from our teaching methods, its sustainability over time, and its generalisability to diverse clinical situations. Are we just teaching students an intellectual understanding of certain concepts, or can such knowledge be translated into not only behavioural skills but also enhanced emotional intelligence that will improve the student's future relationships with patients after qualification? The internalisation and processing of knowledge may also be correlated with the mode of teaching: for example, there is much evidence to show that experiential and active small group learning are among the essential components required to move from just 'knowing about' to knowing how to communicate effectively (Brafman, 2003; Silverman, 2009). In this respect, the design of teaching in both the Student Psychotherapy Scheme and the Balint groups may be particularly potent through the experience of participating in the small group settings of the Balint groups and Student

Psychotherapy Scheme supervision groups, and with the direct and prolonged experience of patient contact in the latter method of learning about the doctor–patient relationship.

Research on the 'student psychotherapist'

Before considering the specific research studies that have been carried out on the UCL Student Psychotherapy Scheme and other schemes based on this model, it is informative to consider some of the wider research surrounding the concept of the medical student as psychotherapist. From the 1950s, American medical schools started offering primary therapist roles to medical students, which became known as the 'student therapist clerkship model' (Oldham et al., 1983). This mode of teaching, in which students took primary responsibility for patients, became popular within undergraduate medical education, as students were thought to learn more than when they were solely passive observers. This was considered particularly important for the surgical and psychiatric specialties in which much of the teaching was considered to be of poor quality. The literature indicates that within psychiatric teaching, the role of the student therapist varied widely between offering the patient some form of psychotherapy with the help of supervision and instruction in psychoanalytic technique, and acting in a less formal role as a case manager. Also, these student interventions were usually fairly short term and offered to patients who had been admitted to inpatient wards (Frank et al., 1987). The extent to which these ideas and innovations in undergraduate teaching in psychiatry received cross-pollination and fertilisation from fellow educators across the Atlantic is not clear, but similar casework by medical students in the teaching of psychiatry is described as early as 1955 at St. Mary's Hospital in London (Davies et al., 1958), which influenced the setting up of the Student Psychotherapy Scheme at UCH shortly afterwards in 1958 (Tredgold, 1962).

From the start, educators were interested in the impact of the student therapist clerkship model on both the students and patients involved. A series of studies examining the attitudes of students and faculty reported that students valued most highly the teaching experiences offering direct patient contact and primary responsibility (Oldham et al., 1983). Moreover, there was evidence that the student therapists could effect positive change in the patients they were treating. One study (Marozas et al., 1971) described an evaluation of symptomatic change in psychiatric patients treated by medical students at Loyola University Stritch School of Medicine in Illinois. The researchers reviewed the records of 50 patients who had been treated by senior medical students under supervision in a psychiatric clinic over a 10-week period. The patients were not selected according to either their diagnosis or potential treatability but assigned to the students solely on the basis of their availability for treatment in the community, on the days when the student was present. Thirty-two of the 50 patients studied reported improvement in symptoms, mostly in the area of disturbance of feelings, particularly anxiety, depression and anger. Patients with a diagnosis of personality disorder showed similar improvement to those diagnosed with what was referred to as 'psychoneurotic reactions'. However, little detail is given of the nature of the treatment delivered by the students, except that it was comprised of weekly half-hour 'treatment interviews'. The study was also limited by the lack of detail regarding symptomatic change recorded in the notes following termination of treatment. Despite this, the authors concluded that medical students were able to effect symptomatic change in the short-term treatment of psychiatric patients.

However, other studies challenged the established superiority of the student therapist clerkship model. Schonfield and Donner (1972) looked at the personality characteristics, style of relating to patients and changes in self-image among students exposed to the psychotherapists' role. The students were classified on the basis of whether they were more 'technique-oriented' or 'patient-oriented'. The experience of being a student psychotherapist was associated with significant negative changes in the technique-oriented students compared to the patient-oriented students. Technique-oriented students became more active, directive, impersonal and distant in their behaviour towards patients. These students also underwent statistically significant negative changes in their perceptions of their patients, none of which occurred among the patient-oriented students. These results prompted the study's authors to call into question the rationale for exposing all students to psychotherapist's role.

Oldham et al. (1983) compared clinical clerkships in psychiatry between students taking on the primary therapist role, and those taking a more traditional participant-observer role. They found no differences between the two groups in the objective assessment of learning of clinical psychiatry (via an exam given to all the students), and found that students preferred the participant-observer role (measured by anonymously surveying their attitudes to their clerkship). They concluded that the participant-observer role was a more appropriate and effective learning experience than the student psycho-therapist role, because conducting psychotherapy was too complex and anxiety provoking for medical students.

Frank et al. (1987) criticised Oldham's conclusion for being based on the students working with very ill patients, as well as the psychotherapy not being conducted by the students as a specific treatment technique. They described an evaluation of a psychiatric clerkship teaching programme at McGill University Medical School in Montreal, Canada, which allowed third- or fourth-year medical students clinical exposure to the conduct of outpatient psychodynamic psychotherapy. This teaching programme formed part of a compulsory 8-week rotation in psychiatry and was comprised of 25 hours per week of didactic teaching seminars, rounds and supervision in traditional areas of a psychiatric clerkship. For the psychodynamic clerkship, the students were given eight didactic lectures on psychodynamic psychotherapy and were assigned a patient referred for short-term therapy. The patients were selected for having a good degree of personality strength, as well as a focal problem for which a psycho-dynamic formulation could be constructed. Patients were excluded if they had severe personality pathology, histories of impulsive, self-harm or suicidal behaviours, psychosis, severe separation difficulties, or the absence of any meaningful relationships. The students met with patients for 10 to 12 sessions over a period of 7 weeks, as well as meeting as a group with their supervisor for 5 hours per week, to go over each session, as well as being introduced to psychoanalytic concepts such as intra-psychic conflict, transference, counter-transference and resistance.

The programme was evaluated in a number of areas. Regarding initial choice of clerkship, it was found that significantly more students opted for the psychotherapy-oriented clerkship than for other psychiatric clerkships, despite showing no significant differences in intended future career choices or preferred professional activities in the two groups. Analysis of students' attitudes following completion of the clerkships showed that students in the psychotherapy-oriented clerkship had significantly more positive attitudes towards the clerkship than students on other clerkships within the rotation. The researchers also showed that students taking this clerkship showed significantly increased skills in taking histories and interacting with medically ill, as well as psychiatric patients, over students taking medical internal medicine clerkships. Finally, follow-up of 806 students in five consecutive classes graduating from McGill Medical School found that the students who took the psychotherapy-oriented clerkship chose psychiatry as a specialty significantly more often than students undergoing rotations elsewhere.

This programme shows striking similarities to the UCL Student Psychotherapy Scheme (which the authors refer to in their paper) and is of relevance in that it appears to be the first description of a North American psychiatric undergraduate clerkship that advocates students seeing care-fully selected outpatients for supervised psychodynamic psychotherapy, albeit for a shorter period than on the UCL scheme. Moreover, the authors found evidence that not only was this programme more popular than other psychiatric clerkships, but that participation improved the student's conduct of the doctor–patient relationship in the non-psychiatric practice of medicine, as well as having a positive influence on psychiatry as a choice of career. As we will see, our own more recent research on the UCL Student Psychotherapy Scheme produced similar outcomes.

Initial research on the UCL and Heidelberg Student Psychotherapy Schemes

Although the UCH Student Psychotherapy Scheme was initiated in 1958, no formal evaluation of its outcomes was conducted until the 1970s, when the Psychosomatic Clinic in the University of Heidelberg set up a similar scheme. The collaboration with German colleagues provided a stimulus to research more scientifically what such schemes might achieve in terms of patient outcomes, as well as looking at why some students opted to join the schemes, whereas others did not (Sturgeon, 1986).

Sturgeon looked at differences and similarities between those students who participated in the UCH scheme and those that didn't. Thirty students who were seeing patients on the scheme and 30 control students who had not participated in the scheme completed questionnaires comprised of items covering biographical data and more open-ended questions about motivations for doing the scheme. He found significant differences between the two groups: the students who joined the scheme were more likely than the controls to express prior interest in psychiatry and psychology, they tended to be older, having done a previous degree or taken time off between school and university, and they were more likely to consider themselves more patient-centred than medicine-centred. By contrast, the students who considered themselves to be more medicine-oriented tended to be less dissatisfied with medicine as a whole and more concerned with academic success than the students in the psychotherapy group. Sturgeon found that the main reason cited by the control group for not opting for the scheme was the time involved.

Sturgeon also found a possible influence of the Student Psychotherapy Scheme on career choice. He contacted 30 students who had done the scheme over a 3-year period and found that ten were already in psychiatry training schemes and two more wished to do psychiatry. This represented over one-third of the students who had done the scheme, which was much more than both the annual proportion of students from UCL at that time who went into psychiatry (9%) and the national average of all medical students choosing psychiatry (4%). However, interpretation of these findings is limited by not knowing whether the students had chosen to do the Student Psychotherapy Scheme because they were already interested in psychiatry as a career, which Sturgeon had demonstrated was more common in students who chose to do the scheme.

At the same time that Sturgeon was conducting his research on the UCH Student Psychotherapy Scheme, the Heidelberg Psychosomatic Clinic were attempting an ambitious evaluation of their own student scheme (Knauss and Senf, 1985). This formed part of a systematic follow-up study that was conducted on all patients in psychotherapy at the clinic between 1978 and 1981 and included a total of 46 patients being treated by 52 medical students under supervision.

The evaluation of the Heidelberg Student Psychotherapy Scheme was divided into two components – a preliminary study and a main study. The preliminary study involved a questionnaire being sent to all the students involved in the scheme asking about their previous interest in psychological problems, previous contact with patients, principal motive for joining the programme and previous practical and theoretical experience in psychotherapy.

The main study included 39 students and 38 patients. For the students this involved a semi-structured follow-up interview conducted by two experienced psychoanalysts with 20 of the students who completed the scheme, and a semi-structured follow-up questionnaire completed by 30 of the 39 students after they had completed the programme. For the patients, the main study involved in-depth psychological interviews by experienced psychoanalysts prior to starting treatment and a 2-year follow-up after finishing therapy, and with further tests at assessment, start of therapy, end of therapy and 2-year follow-up.

The results of the study were impressive. Most of the students considered discussion of their patients in supervision to have been the most rewarding experience of medical school. They found it helpful to discover that their own emotional reactions had an effect on their patient, and to talk in supervision about their anxieties, such as fears of being too inexperienced, fears of failure, feeling angry or sexually aroused by patients, or disappointment at not being able to help every patient. Students who had participated in the scheme and were now doctors felt they had learnt the following skills:

- an ability to recognise and control disturbing experiences, especially anxiety and uncertainty, which helped them create better therapeutic relationships with their patients;
- to be better listeners;
- a recognition of when the patient wanted to talk;
- to feel more relaxed when discussing embarrassing subjects such as sexual problems;
- an increased awareness of the psychological and emotional difficulties of patients and how they linked to their physical illness;
- an ability to handle separations;
- an increased acceptance of their own limitations, and ability to cope with feelings of guilt or hopelessness at not being able to cure, especially in terminally ill patients.

However, the students also reported that they felt they had learnt little from the scheme about working in teams, and found it hard to deal with the distant clinical atmosphere in hospitals that they encountered post-qualification.

The outcomes of patients in the Heidelberg Student Psychotherapy Scheme research were also impressive. The patients were evaluated via a number of methods, including self-reported questionnaires, follow-up interviews with experienced clinicians, and the written reports and interviews of their student therapists. In their follow-up interviews, the interviewing clinicians judged that 87% of the patients had made good or very good progress, around half showed better self-esteem, and around two-thirds showed more independence in social relationships. Only two patients were reported as having deteriorated in any of these areas. Over half of the patients reported that the opportunity to talk to an independent person without judgement had been the most important experience in therapy. There was a high degree of agreement between the students' and patients' assessment of the relationship between them and therapeutic progress.

These favourable subjective findings derived from follow-up interviews with the patients and students, and the students' final reports, were backed by more objective data. All of the patients who completed self-report questionnaires showed significant improvement in a majority of symptoms between the start and finish of therapy, including dizziness, numbness, chest pain and stomach aches. However, this change was not sustained overall at 2-year follow-up. The majority of patients also reported being able to more easily express anger, experienced less anxiety, felt less inhibited with members of the opposite sex and felt less at the mercy of external circumstances at the end of treatment. These changes were sustained at 2-year follow-up.

The authors concluded that patients can be effectively treated by medical students. Positive experiences of the patients included emotional release, their own active participation and the opening up of new areas of experience, which led to symptom improvement, greater self-esteem and improved personal relationships. However, the study is limited in that there were no control groups for either the students or patients, and it is not clear how the results of the interviews were analysed. Nevertheless, the study is valuable in being the only published research that has looked at the outcomes of the patients treated by medical students participating in a Student Psychotherapy Scheme.

Who wants to do psychiatry? The influence of participation in a Student Psychotherapy Scheme on career choice

As we have seen, Sturgeon discovered that a higher proportion than expected of the medical students who participated in the UCL Student Psychotherapy Scheme over a 3-year period chose to train in psychiatry as a speciality following qualification, a finding that was replicated by Frank et al. (1987) in their study of career choice of the students who did the psychodynamically-oriented clerkship. However, in both studies, the lack of control group made it difficult to establish the direction of causality: was it the scheme itself that had a positive influence on the students' choice of psychiatry as a career, or were students who were already interested in psychiatry more likely to opt to participate in the scheme than the students who did not choose to participate? Prompted by concern regarding the longstanding unpopularity of psychiatry among medical students in general, and the difficulties in recruiting enough doctors to psychiatry in the UK and in other countries, we decided to conduct a study that was designed to investigate these questions in a more methodologically robust manner (Yakeley et al., 2004). This involved studying a much larger sample of students to ensure sufficient statistical power, and comparing these to a randomly selected control group.

Following an initial pilot study, we sent questionnaires asking about career choice to 198 subjects and 200 controls. The subject group comprised students for whom we had records as participating in the Student Psychotherapy Scheme over a 10-year period between 1982 and 1992. The control group came from lists of all medical students who had attended the medical school for each of the years between 1982 and 1992 according to the UCL Alumni Relations office. From these lists we randomly chose 200 controls, matched for each year, but who had not participated in the scheme.

In the questionnaire we asked about their current post and choice of career. If the person had chosen to do psychiatry they were asked to complete further questions: whether they had chosen University College Hospital Medical School because they were interested in psychiatry, whether they knew about the Student Psychotherapy Scheme before they came to UCH, and crucially, whether they were considering a career in psychiatry before they became a clinical medical student. If they had participated in the scheme, we asked whether it had been a positive or negative influence on their choice of psychiatry as a career. We also asked what other factors in their medical training had influenced them to do psychiatry. Those subjects and controls who had not chosen psychiatry as a career were asked whether they had considered psychiatry before doing clinical medical studies, and if they had participated in the scheme, whether this had contributed to their decision not to do psychiatry.

Of a total of 398 subjects and controls contacted, 80.7% sent back completed questionnaires. The response rate was significantly higher in the subject group (85.4%) compared to the controls (76.0%). Six 'subjects' replied that they had not participated, leaving a total of 163 subjects who replied and had participated in the scheme.

To determine whether participation in the Student Psychotherapy Scheme influenced the decision to pursue psychiatry as a career after qualification it was necessary to look at the career choices of the students in both groups who had not already considered psychiatry as a career prior to participating in the scheme. Of the 163 subjects, 42 had become psychiatrists (25.8%) compared to only four psychiatrists among the 152 controls (2.6%). Seventy-seven of these 163 participants in the scheme who had sent back the questionnaire had not thought about doing psychiatry before entering the scheme. Of these, 11 had become psychiatrists (14.3%) compared to only two (1.6%) of the 128 controls (of 152 respondents) who had not considered psychiatry as a career at the same stage. This difference is highly significant (P < 0.001).

We were also interested to see if the scheme had dissuaded any of the students from choosing psychiatry as a career. Eleven subjects who had participated recorded that this was the case, although of these, three had become psychiatrists nevertheless. The remaining 39 subjects who had become psychiatrists wrote that participation had positively influenced their decision to do psychiatry, including all 11 who had not considered psychiatry before participating in the scheme.

The most commonly cited other influence that the students in our study reported on their choice of psychiatry as a career was a positive experience of the psychiatric clinical clerkship or 'firm'. Other factors included completing a BSc in psychology, being able to spend more time listening to patients, positive role models from psychiatric teachers, disillusionment with the medical model, and psychiatry being an easier career in which to progress compared to other specialities. A recent study of choice and rejection of psychiatry as a career of UK medical graduates from 1974 to 2009 found that three factors had a greater influence on career choice for psychiatry than on doctor's choice for other clinical careers: the doctors' self-appraisal of their own skills, their inclinations before medical school, and their experience of the subject as a student (Goldacre et al., 2013). Factors that have been cited most frequently in positively influencing choice of psychiatry as a career for the medical student include positive observations of the psychiatrist–patient relationship, emphasis on treating the 'whole person', amount of patient inter-action, giving students clinical responsibility and positive experiences with members of the psychiatric faculty or department (Zimny and Sata, 1986; Ney et al., 1990; Lee et al., 1995; Kirchner and Owen, 1996; Brockington and Mumford, 2002). These are all experiences that are promoted by participation in the Student Psychotherapy Scheme; indeed, one of the main original aims was to enable students to learn in more depth about the doctor–patient rela-tionship in which 'whole-person' or 'patient-centred' medicine is emphasised. Many participants in our study who had not become psychiatrists, in particular those who had become GPs, commented on their returned questionnaires on how useful the scheme had been in understanding the doctor–patient relationship and helping them in their subsequent clinical work.

The influences determining the final choice of career of a medical student are of course complex and multifactorial, and we cannot conclude that partici-pation in the scheme definitively influenced the students to become psy-chiatrists. Our study was limited in that it was a retrospective, not a prospective, study, and allocation to subject and control groups was not randomised. The students' answers to our question as to whether they were interested in pursuing psychiatry as a career prior to joining the scheme may have been influenced by retrospective recall, given that for some of the students we were asking them to remember their thoughts on future career choice from more than 15 years previously. Nevertheless, our study indicates that participation in a Student Psychotherapy Scheme may be a positive influence for medical students choosing psychiatry, and significantly for those who did not have a prior interest in psychiatry before entering medical school. This is an important finding, given the longstanding recruitment crisis in the speciality in many countries, while demand for psychiatric services is increasing. In the USA, 75% of its counties have a shortage of psychiatrists (Thomas et al., 2009), and in the UK, in 2009, 15% of all unfilled consultant posts were in psychiatry (Goldacre et al., 2013). The percentage of newly qualified doctors choosing to do psychiatry as their first choice of career has remained constant for 35 years at only 4%, which is very similar to the percentage of doctors entering psychiatry residency training in the US in recent years (Salsberg et al., 2008).

We also recognise that even if a Student Psychotherapy Scheme encourages medical students to think about psychiatry as a career, it requires considerable expertise and resources, as well as involving complex clinical governance and ethical issues, and will only be available to a small proportion of medical students. One of the reasons that we introduced a different form of psychodynamic teaching about the doctor–patient relationship – Balint groups for medical students – was to be able to offer more students the opportunity for this type of experience. We should therefore be interested in whether participation in Balint groups – which are easier to set up and deliver, and economically more efficient in being potentially available to a large proportion of each medical school year intake – has a positive influence on medical students in their choice of psychiatry as a future career. At the same time, it is also important to remember that the primary aim of both the Student Psychotherapy Scheme and the Balint groups is to teach medical students about emotional and psychodynamic aspects of the doctor–patient relationship based on a whole-person approach, which we hope will facilitate the student in developing attitudes and skills which are of benefit to patients whatever the speciality of the doctor.

Medical student Balint group research

Balint groups have been used as a teaching method for medical students and have been reported in the literature in several countries, including Germany (Paar et al., 1983; Lang, 1988), Austria (Sollner et al., 1992), Italy (Castiglioni and Bellini, 1982), Switzerland (Luban-Plozza, 1989; 1995), South Africa (Levenstein, 1980), Poland (Jugowar and Skommer, 2003), Finland (Torrpa et al., 2008), Sweden (Haggmark and Haggmark, 2005), the United States (Brazeau et al., 1998; Turner, 2005), and more recently Australia (Parker and Leggett, 2012), Brazil (Taveira et al., 2010) and Peru (Mendoza, 2009). Although some of these authors have attempted to evaluate various factors, such as students' motivations for choosing to participate in a Balint group, the content of the Balint group discussions, and the experience and impact on the students, the only rigorous qualitative study that has been conducted to date of a medical student Balint group is that by Torppa et al. (2008).

Thus, Castiglioni and Bellini (1982) described students' motivations for participating in Balint groups. They found that initial motivations included curiosity, use of the group as a complement to a psychiatry course, and the chance to engage in personal analysis. Later motivations reflected the purpose of the group: to provide a chance for affective ripening and to improve the doctor–patient relationship. Paar et al. (1983) looked at the content of discussion of a Balint group of 19 medical students, and found that they were more likely to talk about patient-centred, rather than disease-centred, concerns. Brazeau et al. (1998), in a more extensive study, described the use of a time-limited Balint group experience that 161 third-year medical students had completed during their clerkship in family medicine at New Jersey Medical School during the 1995–1996 academic year. Of the 98 students who completed an evaluation of their experience, two-thirds evaluated the Balint group discussion and effectiveness of the leaders with the highest scores. The authors also reported the topics that recurred most consistently in the Balint group discussions: students feeling angry with or withdrawing from non-compliant patients; irritation at somatising patients; emotional aspects of dealing with death and dying; liking or disliking patients because something about the patient resonated with the student's own personal or family background; reactions to attractive patients and patients who cross professional boundaries; issues specifically related to being a student, e.g. being the lowest in the medical hierarchy; and witnessing inappropriate doctor–patient interactions without being able to intervene. However, each medical student was only offered four Balint groups, each lasting for 1 hour.

Torppa et al. (2008) used a grounded theory-based approach with thematic content analysis of the field notes of the discussions of cases presented in Balint groups for medical students in Helsinki, Finland. They looked at 15 Balint sessions involving nine female students, and identified five triggers for case narrations: witnessing injustice, value conflict, difficult human relationships, incurable patients, and role confusion, that originated from three distinct contexts – patient encounters, confusing experiences in medical education, and tension between privacy and profession. Four main discussion themes were identified: feelings related to patients, building professional identity, negative role models, and cooperation with other medical professionals. The authors concluded that the concept of 'cases' in student Balint groups was wider than in traditional Balint groups. Feelings related to patients and to one's own role as a student doctor were openly discussed in groups. The discussions often touched on professional growth and future professional identity as doctors. However, this study was limited by its small sample size, and being a solely female group.

Recent research on the UCL medical student Balint groups and the Student Psychotherapy Scheme

Following the introduction of Balint groups for medical students at UCL in 2004, we became interested in building on what was already known about Balint groups for medical students from these studies in other countries, by researching in more detail what their impact might be on medical student learning in comparison with the impact on students of the Student Psychotherapy Scheme.

In a preliminary qualitative study, Suckling (2005) reviewed three separate groups that she had conducted and made notes on shortly after each group session. Of a total of 63 patient cases presented by the students, she identified 17 main themes of discussion, of which the following 10 were most common: the students' role, confidentiality, consent, the very ill patient, death and dying, revulsion towards patients, history taking, professional boundaries, the student–patient relationship, and the doctors' behaviour. These themes are very similar to those reported as being most frequently brought up by students in the studies by Brazeau et al. (1998) and Torppa et al. (2008) described above. Suckling also analysed the feedback forms filled in by the students after they had completed the course of Balint groups, and found that students reported that participation in the Balint group meetings increased their confidence, improved their communication skills, encouraged whole-patient medicine, encouraged reflection, provided support and increased their enjoyment of their work. This is described in greater detail in Chapter 5.

This qualitative research is informative, but we were also interested in conducting more quantitative outcome research – by means of a randomised controlled trial – to evaluate the effectiveness of our two psychodynamic psychotherapy teaching methods, the Student Psychotherapy Scheme and the Balint groups, in teaching first-year clinical medical students about doctor–patient communication and the doctor–patient relationship. The use of a control group comprised of medical students who did not participate in either of the teaching interventions was necessary to determine whether any changes observed might have been attributed to the teaching interventions, rather than to confounding factors such as other teaching that the students were exposed to.

The only other published study to date using the methodology of a randomised controlled trial to evaluate the effectiveness of a Student Psychotherapy Scheme is that of Shapiro et al. (2009) in their evaluation of a communication skills programme for first-year medical students at the University of Toronto. This programme was set up in 1995 and explicitly modelled on the UCH Student Psychotherapy Scheme in offering medical students the opportunity to meet weekly with carefully selected outpatients on a one-to-one basis for 4 months while receiving supervision from a faculty psychiatrist. In their study, students over 4 consecutive academic years were randomly allocated either to a group who received this educational intervention or a waiting list control group, yielding 38 intervention participants and 41 control participants. The assessment instruments, which were administered at baseline, 4 and 8 months, comprised a self-assessment questionnaire of the participants' interpersonal competence; ratings of the participants interviewing two standardised patients using the Interpersonal Skills Rating Scale (ISRS, Schnabel et al., 1991); and assessment of the students' expressed empathy using the Staff–Patient Interaction Rating Scale (SPIR, Gallop et al., 1990), which is a questionnaire inviting open-ended responses to questions made by hypothetical patients and rated by trained external raters according to a manual. However, the results of the study were inconclusive, with only the SPIR showing a significantly increased improvement over time compared to the control group, so only partially supporting the hypothesis that the programme improved students' communication skills. However, students' ratings of their interpersonal competence significantly decreased over time, suggesting that either the intervention was detrimental to the students' ability to communicate therapeutically, or that students' self-evaluation of their communication skills is an ineffective measure of actual performance.

For our study (Yakeley et al., 2011), we randomised 30 students from the same intake from the academic year 2006–2007 to three groups, each containing ten students. All of the students had originally attended our annual introductory lecture about the two schemes and had then been interviewed to assess their suitability to see psychotherapy patients. The first group was for students to do the Student Psychotherapy Scheme for 1 year between January 2006 and January 2007. The second group was for students to participate in a Balint group which ran for 3 months between January and April 2006. The third group was a Balint group which ran for 3 months between April and June 2006. This last group acted as a partial control, in that at 3 months, these students had not received any teaching compared to those randomly allocated to the other two groups. We decided not to have a pure control group, as all of the students volunteering for the research had opted to do the Student Psychotherapy Scheme or a Balint group for their Student Selected Component (SSC). Both Balint groups were run by the same two group leaders to avoid any variation in the style of the group leaders which might have interfered with comparisons between groups 2 and 3.

Because we could not find a suitable pre-existing validated measure that tested knowledge of emotional aspects of the doctor–patient relationship we designed our own measure. This was a qualitative questionnaire that asked a series of questions about the emotional aspects of the doctor–patient relationship (see Appendix 1). The questionnaire aimed to ascertain that the student had become aware of the significance of the relationship between the doctor/student and patient, that the student recognised the feelings which were evoked by the interaction with the patient and was able to use these for the benefit of the patient, that the student could be aware of the emotional meanings of the patient's physical symptoms, and that the student was aware of his or her own limitations.

We administered this questionnaire at three separate time points: at baseline, before the students received any teaching; at 3 months; and at 1 year. The questionnaires were marked by three independent raters, according to a set of 'ideal answers' (see Appendix 2) that we had compiled. Shortly after the research started, two students dropped out of group 1, one due to illness, and the other as she decided that she could not commit to participating in the Student Psychotherapy Scheme after all. This left eight students in group 1, ten in group 2 and ten in group 3.

The main findings were (a) a significant improvement in the scores compared to baseline scores in all three groups at 1 year, after the students had all participated in one of the two teaching methods, and (b) at 3 months, a trend, that did not quite reach significance, towards higher scores in groups 1 and 2, containing students who had participated in the SPS and Balint groups respectively, compared to those in the control group (group 3) who had not participated in either intervention at that stage. These results supported our hypothesis in suggesting that the interventions were effective in increasing students' knowledge of the doctor–patient relationship compared to students who did not receive these teaching experiences.

There were various limitations to our study. There was no control group at 1 year, and also no significant difference between the scores of all three groups at the end of the study. We therefore cannot confidently assume that the significant improvements in the students' scores at 1 year compared to their scores at the beginning were due to the effects of the Student Psychotherapy Scheme or Balint groups, and not due to other influences that they may have been subject to during their first year of clinical medical studies.

An alternative explanation for the significant increase in scores in all the groups in our study at 1 year could be a maturation in the personalities of the students over time, independent of the effects of any teaching programme. However, such a hypothesis is not supported by the many studies which show evidence of a diminution of communication skills, patient-centred attitudes and empathy in medical students as they progress through medical school without some formal input. This has been attributed to the dominant medical culture promoting biomedical mechanisms of disease rather than psychosocial determinants (Haidet et al., 2002; Nogueira-Martins et al., 2006; Tsimtsiou et al., 2007; Shapiro, 2008). Students may lose their idealism and lose their wish to help others and become disillusioned and cynical, resulting in coping mechanisms of distance and detachment at the expense of awareness of patients' concerns and emotions. This may have accounted for an interesting result in our study, which was a decrease in scores from baseline to 3 months in the partial control group of students who had as yet received no intervention.

Another limitation of our study was the small number of students involved overall, which was determined by the limited number of places that we had available on the Student Psychotherapy Scheme. We also had a poor response rate at 3 months, which may have been due to students' reluctance to fill out the same questionnaire that they had only completed 3 months before.

We also did not use a pre-existing validated measure of communication skills, but devised our own measure. Most measures of communication skills require trained raters to assess video-taped interactions between students and actors or 'standardised' patients, which are costly, time consuming, and often have poor inter-rater reliability (Lurie et al., 2008). Moreover, emotional communications are difficult to measure in simulated scenarios. Existing measures of empathy, emotional intelligence and patient-centred attitudes such as the Bar-One Emotional Quotient (EQ-i) (Fletcher et al., 2009), the Patient Practitioner Orientation Scale (PPOS) (Humphris and Kaney, 2001; Nogueira-Martins et al., 2006) and the Doctor–Patient Communication Inventory (DPCI) (Schneider and Tucker, 1992) have been used to test medical students, but these instruments do not address knowledge of the doctor–patient relationship from a psychodynamic viewpoint, which we felt was an important aspect of our teaching methods. We therefore attempted to create a questionnaire that tested the students' knowledge of psychodynamic and emotional contributions to the doctor–patient relationship, for example, their understanding of the unconscious processes involved in emotional communication, or the importance of a patient's prior attachment experiences in influencing their relationship to the doctor. However, our questionnaire may only have tested their knowledge at an intellectual level, and we do not know whether or how such acquired knowledge translates into actual behavioural change in the form of improved communication skills with patients. Furthermore, our ideal answers to the questionnaire may also have assumed a greater potential in the students for learning about the doctor–patient relationship than was possible with so short an exposure to these psychodynamic teaching approaches, and may explain why the changes in the three groups were relatively small.

Finally, the inter-rater reliability between our raters in the study was not perfect, with the observers having different overall mean scores, and less than ideal correlation between the scores.

Nevertheless, we believe this is the first reported randomised controlled trial evaluating a Student Psychotherapy Scheme and Balint groups for medical students, and our questionnaire is currently being used to evaluate another Student Psychotherapy Scheme (Martucci, personal communication, 2011) and in Balint groups for core psychiatry trainees (Shaikh, personal communication, 2013). Previous studies have shown that students' acquisition of knowledge of communication skills may be optimised when communication training is given with supervised patient contact (Baerheim et al., 2007). Moreover, a meta-analysis of studies of 24 randomised controlled trials evaluating the effects of teaching interventions on medical students' patient communication skills showed that the two most effective teaching methods in improving student performance were direct feedback on a student–patient interview and small group discussions (Smith et al., 2007). Both of our teaching methods combine all of these methods: supervised patient contact, small group discussion, and detailed feedback on student–patient interactions from either the student's supervisor in the case of the Student Psychotherapy Scheme, or from the Balint group leaders.

Future directions

If we wish to encourage other educators and clinicians to implement similar methods to teach medical students about the role of emotions in illness and psychodynamic approach to the doctor–patient relationship and clinical communication, we need to provide evidence of their benefits. I have summarised the research that has been conducted to date, both at our own medical school in the UK and at medical schools in other countries, on the impact of medical student participation in Student Psychotherapy Schemes and Balint groups. These studies have shown several significant objective outcomes for the students involved, including increased knowledge of the doctor–patient relationship and influence on career choice. These findings should be considered in the context of the wider body of research that demonstrates that a positive therapeutic relationship between doctor and patient, and particularly one in which the role of emotions is acknowledged and understood, is associated with improved patient care and safety at many levels.

We need to continue to develop new tools to demonstrate the outcomes and efficacy of our teaching methods, combined with qualitative methods to understand the processes involved, as well as evaluating the experience of the students. One key area of future study will be to elucidate in more detail how students learn to enhance their empathic understanding of patients, to reflect on their own and their patients' emotions, how this translates into effective clinical behaviours, and how we can accurately and reliably assess these acquired attitudes and skills. Reflective practice, which includes personal self-awareness, dealing with uncertainty, and recognising boundaries, is recognised as one of the overriding principles governing all areas of medical practice, including the undergraduate curriculum (von Fragstein et al., 2008).

Other ways to promote more sustained learning, such as giving students more responsibility for patients, continues to be recognised as important in consolidating knowledge, as well as allowing for an appreciation of the different perspectives that patients, carers, doctors and other professionals may have on physical and mental illness and their management (Thomson and Dave, 2011). However, such responsibility usually entails giving the medical student tasks such as summarising case notes, taking a history, interviewing carers or conducting mental state examinations, and it is now rare for students to be allowed to have a more direct role in the patient's treatment as occurs in a Student Psychotherapy Scheme. This shift away from the 'student therapist' model may be the result of the increasing concern for patient safety and the introduction of simulation techniques in medical training.

Conducting methodologically sound research, however, requires considerable expertise and resources, and it is therefore advantageous to link up with others interested in the field. To this end, we are fortunate in currently joining forces with colleagues at Bristol Medical School and King's College London

Medical School to continue researching our respective Student Psychotherapy Schemes, as well as collaborating with others who are involved in the setting up and running of medical student Balint groups in Sheffield, Leeds and Nottingham in the UK (Johnston, personal communication, 2013) and in Melbourne, Sydney and Woolangong in Australia with the aim of disseminating the patient-centred teaching approach that Balint founded over 40 years ago.

Note

1   Balint thanks Professor Millar of the University of Aberdeen for suggesting this term to him (Balint et al., 1969). Enid Balint also speaks of 'patient-centred medicine' in a paper published in 1969 (E. Balint, 1969).

Appendix 1

Questionnaire about the doctor–patient relationship

1   What effect can the relationship between a doctor/student and patient have on the patient's overall care?
2   How may a doctor's/student's feelings be affected by a patient?
3   How may a doctor/student use those feelings in relation to the patient?
4   How do you cope with your anxiety and uncertainty in your work with patients?
5   Do you feel that the relationship between the doctor/student and the patient should be an equal one? If not, why?
6   Why is it important to understand the nature of the patient's attachment to the doctor/student?
7   How do you recognise emotion in a patient when it is not verbalised?
8   Please comment on your experience in this project.

Appendix 2

Guide to marking questionnaire about the doctor–patient relationship

The following is a guide to marking the students' questionnaires.
   For each question score out of a total of 3.

   0 = completely incorrect answer;
   1 = partially right answer;
   2 = completely correct answer;
   3 = exceptional/original and correct answer.

An 'ideal' answer should include reference to all of the following ideas for each question.

1 What effect can the relationship between a doctor/student and patient have on the patient's overall care?

A good relationship can promote trust between the doctor/student and patient which will:

(a) Allow the patient to confide in the doctor/patient and so give them a fuller history.
(b) Help the patient to comply with treatment given.
(c) May help the patient to recover from their illness, because the mind and body of the patient are taken into account, and affect each other. If the patient feels understood and contained by the doctor, this may improve the patient's mental state, which can have a positive effect on the patient's overall physical and psychological health. If the relationship is a poor one, it can have a very negative effect on patient care.

2 How may a doctor's/student's feelings be affected by a patient?

(a) The doctor/student may identify with the patient's feelings and so experience the emotions the patient is experiencing, e.g. the helplessness or despair of the patient is experienced by the doctor/student. This may be because the patient's feelings and experiences may resonate with previous experiences of the doctor/student. If the doctor/student does identify with the patient's problems, and does not recognise this, they may be less able to help the patient.
(b) The doctor/student may be the recipient of the patient's projections and so experience negative or positive emotions that belong to past relationships in the patient's childhood with significant figures like parents. If the projections are taken personally, this may affect treatment.
(c) It may be difficult to recognise the above (i.e. (b)), but the doctor/student may be aided in this by developing self-knowledge and sensitivity to his/her own experiences and how they have affected him/her emotionally. This may be pointed out by supervisors.

3 How may a doctor/student use those feelings in relation to the patient?

(a) These feelings can help him or her to better understand the patient and so be more empathic. They can use these by acknowledging them, which can help deepen rapport, e.g. 'I can see you are feeling very angry, but I'm not quite sure what it's about. Can we talk about it?'
(b) By recognising the patient's positive and negative emotions, especially when these are projected onto them, the doctor/student may better understand their own emotional reactions to the patient.

(c) The doctor/student's emotional reactions to the patient may be similar to feelings that the patient evokes in other people, recognition of which can help the doctor/student understand in more detail the interpersonal relationships and effects on others the patient may have (e.g. in patients who present as hostile).

(d) The doctor/student may recognise that the patient may be experiencing others in ways based on their previous experiences with significant others. For example, the patient may experience the doctor as a critical parent, and respond in a hostile way.

4 How do you cope with your anxiety and uncertainty in your work with patients?

(a) Acknowledge that I can sometimes feel anxious or uncertain.
(b) By trying to reflect on why I am anxious or uncertain.
(c) By discussing these feelings with a senior colleague.

5 Do you feel that the relationship between the doctor/student and the patient should be an equal one? If not, why?

(a) Although the doctor should respect the ideas and views of the patient, and try to understand their social and cultural context as well as their personal history, the relationship between doctor and patient cannot be an equal relationship.

(b) Whereas a patient comes to a doctor/student for help with physical and/or psychological symptoms and distress and can expect help and understanding, a doctor/student should not impose his own difficulties on the patient.

(c) The doctor/student can expect that many patients will develop a significant attachment to their doctor/student which gives rise to dependency on the doctor/student. This attachment may be based on the patient's previous experiences and attachment/relationship history with significant others.

(d) The reverse may happen in that the student/doctor may come to depend upon the patient to make them feel good about themselves.

6 Why is it important to understand the nature of the patient's attachment to the doctor/student?

(a) The nature of the attachment can throw light on past significant attachments and so will help the doctor/student to better appreciate the meaning of the patient's negative and positive reactions to him or her and so facilitate the development of a more caring relationship.

(b) For example, patients who have had a disrupted attachment history, who may have experienced a parent's death or been in care, may become very attached to caring authority figures such as the doctor and their condition may deteriorate when that doctor leaves. It is important to recognise and understand this.

(c) The relationship the patient develops with the doctor may also tell the doctor something about the patient's current interpersonal relationships with their family and friends, which may give useful information regarding their current social functioning and level of support.

7 How do you recognise emotion in a patient when it is not verbalised?

(a) By studying their facial expression and other bodily gestures, as well as their self-care.

(b) By studying the emotions they arouse in the doctor/student. These may be emotions that are difficult for the patient to tolerate and acknowledge consciously, e.g. feelings of anger or sadness, that are then unconsciously projected by the patient onto the doctor/student, who experiences them instead.

Conclusion

Peter Shoenberg

One student wrote about her psychotherapy with a patient with unexplained medical symptoms:

> The problems that Jenny was experiencing with her bladder and her bowels were a constant theme during the psychotherapy. In the first few sessions she spoke almost exclusively about them. I thought that they were safe topics she could discuss, as I was a medical student, when other things were too difficult. Her symptoms were of recurrent urinary tract infections and bowel problems associated with pelvic floor and lower back muscle tightening and pain. She also suffered with headaches and lethargy. Jenny was initially reluctant to think that her symptoms were linked to her feelings or emotions … However, by looking at examples of how the mind can affect the body and vice versa, such as the migraine she always got on returning from her parents' house or the strange mood she felt during her periods, she was able to see that her mood did affect her symptoms. For example, she had fewer urinary tract infections whilst feeling happy compared with when she was feeling low.
>
> We explored the significance of her symptoms. She remembered that as a child at school she had been very anxious about not making it to the toilet on time, fearing that she would have an accident in the classroom. As a result, she often spent much of break-time sitting on the toilet, making sure she went to the toilet just before the school bell rang, so as to ensure there would be no subsequent accidents in the classroom. At home she had been taught that to use the toilet was dirty and in some way wrong and should never be discussed. This was similar to the way in which emotions were treated at home: we now explored the link between the use of the toilet and her expression of her emotions and I wondered if sometimes the toilet was her way to express these feelings. Although she claimed not to understand how this might be, she gained insight into the way she expressed her emotions and eventually could interpret new symptoms in this light. For example, when trying to express her feelings about the ending of the

therapy, she developed a cough that interrupted her: she now interpreted this as meaning that she did not want to discuss her feelings about this forthcoming ending which would be so difficult for her.

As we discussed the end of the therapy, she compared it to an antibiotic, by which she meant that she thought it would continue to have an effect after it had ended. This was interesting for me, as it showed her ability to link the medical and emotional side of her complaints to the medical and emotional side of me, a medical student and her psychotherapist. It appeared that I had come to symbolize and indeed replace the antibiotics on which Jenny had been so dependent, when we had first begun the psychotherapy.

(Sallnow, personal communication, in Shoenberg, *Psychosomatics. The Uses of Psychotherapy*, 2007, pp. 203–4).

In this short extract from one student's work with a patient we can see the importance of the journey she and her patient made in this year of therapy, from a disease-oriented understanding of the patient's condition to one based on a mutual appreciation of the patient's underlying emotions. The chapters in this book bear witness to many such journeys made by students and their patients, either in the Student Psychotherapy Scheme or in the Balint groups and the ways in which we as psychotherapists can help them to make the best use of their emotional experiences. Such teaching experiences are rewarding for all concerned: teacher, student and patient. For us as teachers, our students' experiences touch off memories of being a medical student that allow us to better identify with our students' difficulties.

Our book is not only a plea for other psychotherapists to encourage their students to make such journeys, but it is also addressed to all medical teachers and their students. Students enter their medical training with an idealism and concern for patients that can easily be lost in the course of their studies. At a time of economic crisis, when so much emphasis is placed on improving the efficiency of health care delivery, there is an even greater need for doctors not to lose sight of their relationship to their patients. Such good relating requires an accurate understanding, not only of the patient's feelings, but also of the feelings he or she arouses in the doctor. We know that as doctors we can spend a lifetime learning to recognise and understand these emotions, so it is vital we are given the chance to begin this process at an early stage of our training.

References

Ahluwalia, S., Murray, E., Stevenson, F., Kerr, C. & Burns, J. (2010) 'A heartbeat moment': Qualitative study of GP views of patients bringing health information from the Internet to a consultation. *British Journal of General Practice*, 60, 88–94.

Antonelou, M. (2010) An account of my student–patient relationship involving the Student Psychotherapy Scheme. In E.R. Petzold and H. Otten (Eds), *The Student, the Patient and the Illness: Ascona Balint Award Essays*. xlibri.de, pp. 22–37.

Baerheim, A., Hjortdahl, P., Holen, A., Anvik, T., Fasmer, O.B., Grimsted, H., Gude, T., Risberg, T. & Vaglum, P. (2007) Curriculum factors influencing knowledge of communication skills among medical students. *BMC Medical Education*, 7, 35.

Balint, E. (1969) The possibilities of patient-centred medicine. *Journal of the Royal College of General Practitioners*, 17, 269–276.

Balint, E., Courtenay, M., Elder, A., Hull, S. & Julian, P. (1993) *The Doctor, the Patient and the Group. Balint Revisited*. London: Routledge.

Balint, M. (1964) *The Doctor, His Patient and the Illness* (2nd edn). London: Pitman Paperbacks.

Balint, M., Ball, D.H. & Hare, M.I. (1969) Training medical students in patient-centred medicine. *Comprehensive Psychiatry*, 10, 249–258.

Ball, D.H. & Wolff, H.H. (1963) An experiment in the teaching of psychotherapy to medical students. *Lancet*, 1, 214–17.

Bateman, A., Brown, D. & Pedder, D. (2010) *Introduction to Psychotherapy* (4th edn). London: Routledge.

Beca, I.J.P., Browne, L.F., Repetto, L.P., Ortiz, P.A. & Salas, A.C. (2007) *Medical Student–Patient Relationship. The Student's Perspective* (in Spanish). *Revista Medica de Chilea*, 135, 1503–1509.

Becker, H. & Knauss, W. (1983) Organisation of the Student Psychotherapy Scheme in Heidelberg. In H.H. Wolff, W. Knauss & W. Brautigam (Eds), *First Steps in Psychotherapy*. Berlin: Springer-Verlag, pp. 34–44.

Beckman, H.B. & Frankel R.M. (1984) The effect of physician behaviour on the collection of data. *Annals of Internal Medicine*, 101, 692–698.

Benbassat, J. & Baumal, R. (2001) Teaching doctor–patient interviewing skills using an integrated learner and teacher-centred approach. *American Journal of Medical Science*, 322, 349–357.

Benbasset, J. & Baumal, R. (2005) Enhancing self-awareness in medical students: an overview of teaching approaches. *Academic Medicine*, 80, 156–161.

Bombeke, K., Symons, L., Debaene, L., De Winter, B., Schol, S. & Van Royen, P. (2010) Help, I'm losing patient-centredness! Experiences of medical students and their teachers. *Medical Education*, 44, 662–673.

Bower, D.J., Young, S., Larson, G., Simpson, D., Tipnis, S., Begaz, T. & Webb, T. (2009) Characteristics of patient encounters that challenge medical students' provision of patient-centered care. *Academic Medicine*, 84 (10 Suppl), S74–78.

Brafman, A. (2003) Memorizing vs Understanding. *Psychoanalytic Psychotherapy*, 17, 119–137.

Brazeau, C.M.L.R., Boyd, L., Rovi, S. & Tesar, C.M. (1998) A one-year experience in the use of Balint groups with third-year medical students. *Families, Systems and Health*, 16, 431–436.

British Medical Association (2003) *Communication skills education for doctors: a discussion document*. London: British Medical Association.

Brockington, I. & Mumford, D. (2002) Recruitment into psychiatry. *British Journal of Psychiatry*, 180, 307–312.

Brown, S. & Gunderman, R.B. (2006) Viewpoint: Enhancing the professional fulfillment of physicians. *Academic Medicine*, 81, 577–582.

Buckman, R., Tulsky, J.A. & Rodin, G. (2011) Empathic responses in clinical practice: intuition or tuition? *Canadian Medical Association Journal*, 183, 569–571.

Bunting, R.F., Benton, J. & Morgan, W.D. (1998) Practical risk management for physicians. *Journal of Health Risk Management*, 18, 29–53.

Canada, A.L., Murphy, P.E., Fitchett, G., et al. (2008) A 3-factor model for FACIT-Sp. *Psychooncology*, 17, 908–916.

Castiglioni, R. & Bellini, M. (1982) The psychological training of medical students using Balint's method: analysis of motivations for the group experience. *Medicina Psicosomatica*, 27, 411–419.

Clark, D. (2007) From margins to centre: a review of the history of palliative care in cancer. *Lancet Oncology*, 8, 430–438.

Clifford, G.J. (1986) A medical student's experience of dynamic psychotherapy with a young woman suffering from asthma. In J.H. Lacey & D.A. Sturgeon (Eds), *Proceedings of the 15th European Conference on Psychosomatic Research*. London: John Libbey, pp 366–368.

Cooper, S., Dogra, N., Lunn, B. & Wright, B. (2011) Undergraduate psychiatry teaching: the core curriculum. In T. Brown & J. Eagles (Eds), *Teaching psychiatry to undergraduates* London: Royal College of Psychiatrists, pp. 26–37.

Coulehan, J. & Williams, P.C. (2001) Vanquishing virtue: the impact of medical education. *Academic Medicine,* 76, 598–605.

Crisp, A.H. (1986). Undergraduate training for communication in medical practice. *Journal of the Royal Society of Medicine*, 79, 568–574.

Curran, L. (2011) What is the role of a medical student in the care of patients? *Journal of the Balint Society*, 39, 26–28.

DasGupta, S. & Charon, R. (2004) Personal illness narratives: using reflective writing to teach empathy. *Academic Medicine*, 79, 351–356.

Davies, T.T., Davies, E.T.L. & O'Neill, D. (1958) Case-work in the teaching of psychiatry. *The Lancet*, 272 (7036), 34–37.

Department of Health (2003) *Statement of guiding principles relating to the commissioning and provision of communication skills training in pre-registration and undergraduate education for healthcare professionals*. London: Department of Health.

Department of Health (2004) *Medical schools: delivering doctors of the future.* London: Department of Health.

Drees, A. & Schwartz, I. (1990) Sensual-imaginative training methods for students of medicine. *Pychotherapy and Psychosomatics*, 53, 68–74.

Faden, R.R., Becker, C., Lewis, C., Freeman, J. & Faden, A.I. (1981) Disclosure of information to patients in medical care. *Medical Care*, 19, 718–733.

Fletcher, I., Leadbetter, P., Curran, A. & O'Sullivan, H. (2009) A pilot study assessing emotional intelligence training and communication skills with 3rd year medical students. *Patient Education and Counseling*, 76, 376–379.

Frances, V., Korsch, B.M. & Morris, M.J. (1969) Gaps in doctor patient communication: patient response to medical advice. *New England Journal of Medicine*, 280, 535–540.

Frank, D., Propst, A. & Goldhamer, P.E. (1987) The effects of teaching medical students psychotherapy skills in the out-patient department. *Canadian Journal of Psychiatry*, 32, 185–189.

Fraser, S.W. & Greenhalgh, T. (2001) Coping with complexity: educating for capability. *British Medical Journal*, 323, 799–803.

Freeling, P., Rao, B.M., Paykel, E.S., Sireling, L.I. & Burton, R.H. (1985) Unrecognised depression in general practice. *British Medical Journal*, 290, 1880–1883.

Gallop, R., Lancee, W.J. & Garfinkel, P.E. (1990) The empathic process and its mediators. A heuristic model. *Journal of Nervous and Mental Disease*, 178, 649–654.

Garner, P. (1981) Psychotherapy: experiences of medical students. *British Medical Journal*, 280, 797–798.

Garner, P. (1985) Psychotherapy: experience as a medical student at UCH. In H.H. Wolff, W. Knauss & W. Brautigam (Eds), *First steps in psychotherapy*. Berlin: Springer-Verlag, pp. 91–94.

Garner, P., Hampson, M. & Prince, S. (1985) Examples and comments by three students of their experience with patients at UCH, London. In H.H. Wolff, W. Knauss & W. Brautigam (Eds), *First steps in psychotherapy*. Berlin: Springer-Verlag, pp. 90–99.

Gazmararian, J.A., Ziemer, D.C. & Barnes, C. (2009) Perception of barriers to self-care management among diabetic patients. *Diabetes Education*, 35, 778–788.

General Medical Council (2002) *Tomorrow's doctors: recommendations on undergraduate medical education*. London: General Medical Council.

Goldacre, M.J., Fazel, S., Smith, F. & Lambert, T. (2013) Choice and rejection of psychiatry as a career: surveys of UK medical graduates from 1974 to 2009. *British Journal of Psychiatry*, 202, 228–234.

Hafferty, F.W. (1998) Beyond curriculum reform: confronting medicine's hidden curriculum. *Academic Medicine*, 73, 403–407.

Haggmark, A. & Haggmark, A. (2005) An exceptional possibility or a mission impossible. International Balint Conference of the Romanian Balint Society.

Haidet, P., Dains, J.E., Paterniti, D.A., Hechtel, L., Chang, T., Tseng, E. & Rogers, J.C. (2002) Medical student attitudes toward the doctor–patient relationship. *Medical Education*, 36, 568–574.

Hampson, M. (1985) Experience gained from the psychotherapy supervision scheme. In H.H. Wolff, W. Knauss & W. Brautigam (Eds), *First Steps in Psychotherapy*. Berlin: Springer-Verlag, pp. 94–96.

Heinonen, E., Lindfors, O., Laaksonen, M.A. & Knekt, P. (2012) Therapists' professional and personal characteristics as predictors of outcome in short- and long-term psychotherapy. *Journal of Affective Disorders*, 138, 301–312.

Helfer, R.E. (1970) An objective comparison of the paediatric interviewing skills of freshman and senior medical students. *Paediatrics*, 45, 623–627.

Hoffman, M. (2000) *Empathy and Moral Development: Implications for Caring and Justice*. New York: Cambridge University Press.

Hojat, M. (2009) Ten approaches for enhancing empathy in health and human services culture. *Journal of Health and Human Services Administration*, 31, 412–450.

Hojat, M., Vergare, M.J., Maxwell, K., Brainard, G., Herrine, S.K., Isenberg, G.A., Veloski, J. & Gonella, J.S. (2009) The devil is in the third year: a longitudinal study of erosion of empathy in medical school. *Academic Medicine*, 84, 1182–1191.

Hoy, L. (2002) Personal view: it's good to talk. *British Medical Journal*, 324, 57.

Hulsker, C. (2004) A student patient relationship in therapeutic setting. *Journal of the Balint Society*, 32, 45.

Humphris, G.M. & Kaney, S. (2001) Assessing the development of communication skills in undergraduate medical students. *Medical Education*, 35, 225–231.

Isen, A.M., Rosenzweig, A.S. & Young, M.J. (1991) The influence of positive affect on clinical problem solving. *Medical Decision Making*, 11, 221–227.

Jugowar, B. & Skommer, M. (2003) The effectiveness of Balint training for medical students. In J. Salinsky & H. Owen (Eds), *The Doctor, the Patient and their Wellbeing – World Wide Proceedings of the 13th International Balint Congress*. Berlin: Ruckzuckdruck, pp. 104–108.

Kataoka, H., Koide, N., Ochi, K., Hojat, M. & Gonella, J.S. (2009) Measurement of empathy among Japanese medical students: psychometrics and score differences by gender and level of medical education. *Academic Medicine*, 84, 1192–1197.

Kaufman, D.M. & Mann, K.V. (2007) *Teaching and learning in medical education: how theory can inform practice*. Edinburgh: Association for the Study of Medical Education.

Kay, J. (1990) Traumatic deidealization and future of medicine. *Journal of the American Medical Association*, 263, 572–573.

King's College London (2012) KCLSoM Student Psychotherapist Scheme. www.kcl.ac.uk/iop/depts/pm/research/sscpr/KCLSoM.aspx

Kirchner, J.E. & Owen, R.R. (1996) Choosing a career in psychiatry. *American Journal of Psychiatry*, 153, 1372.

Knauss, W. & Senf, W. (1985) Follow-up results of the student psychotherapy project in Heidelberg. In H.H. Wolff, W. Knauss & W. Brautigam (Eds), *First Steps in Psychotherapy*. Berlin: Springer-Verlag, pp. 65–76.

Korszun, A., Dinos, S., Ahmed, K. & Bhui, K. (2012) Medical student attitudes about mental illness: does medical school education reduce stigma? *Academic Psychiatry*, 36, 197–204.

Kramer, D., Ber, R. & Moore, M. (1987) Impact of workshop on students' and physicians' rejecting behaviours in patient interviews. *Journal of Medical Education*, 62, 904 –910.

Kurlander, J.E., Kerr, E.A., Krein, S., Heisler, M. & Piette, J.D. (2009) Cost-related non adherence to medications among patients with diabetes and chronic pain: factors beyond finances. *Diabetes Care*, 32, 2143–2148.

Kurtz, S., Silverman, J. & Draper, J. (2005) *Teaching and Learning Communication Skills in Medicine* (2nd edn). Oxford: Radcliffe Publishing Ltd.

Lang, H. (1988) The use of the Balint group method in teaching medical psychology, psychosomatic medicine, and psychotherapy to medical students. *Psychologie Medicale*, 20, 2045–2047.

Launer, J., Blake, S. & Daws, D. (Eds) (2005) *Reflecting on Reality: Psychotherapists at Work in Primary Care*. Tavistock Clinic Series. London: Karnac.

Lee, E.K., Kaltreider, N. & Crouch, J. (1995) Pilot study of current factors influencing the choice of psychiatry as a specialty. *American Journal of Psychiatry*, 152, 1066–1069.

Levenstein, S. (1980) An undergraduate Balint group in Cape Town. *South African Medical Journal*, 62, 89–90.

Lo, C., Zimmermann, C., Gagliese, L., Li, M. & Rodin, G. (2011) Sources of spiritual well-being in advanced cancer. *British Medical Journal Supportive and Palliative Care*, 1, 149–153.

Luban-Plozza, B. (1989) A new training method – 20 years of student Balint groups. *Shweizerische Rundschau für Medizin Praxis*, 78, 1192–1196.

Luban-Plozza, B. (1995) Empowerment techniques: from doctor-centred (Balint approach) to patient-centred discussion groups. *Patient Education and Counseling*, 26, 257–263.

Lurie, S.J., Mooney, C.J., Nofziger, A.C., Meldrum, S.C. & Epstein, R.M. (2008) Further challenges in measuring communication skills: accounting for actor effects in standardized patient assessments. *Medical Education*, 42, 662–668.

Mackillop, W.J., Stewart, W.E., Ginsberg, A.D. & Stewart, S.S. (1988) Cancer patients' perceptions of their disease and its treatment. *British Journal of Cancer*, 58, 355–358.

MacLeod, R. (1991) *Patients with advanced breast cancer: the nature and disclosure of their concerns (dissertation)*. Manchester: Manchester University.

Malan, D. (1999) *Individual Psychotherapy and the Science of Psychodynamics* (2nd edn). Oxford: Butterworth-Heinemann.

Marozas, R.J., Huncke, P.J. & Bohnert, P.J. (1971) Evaluation of symptomatic change in psychiatric patients treated by medical students. *Journal of Medical Education*, 46, 889–895.

Martin, D.P., Gilson, B.S., Bergner, M., Bobbit, R.A., Pollard, W.E., Conn, J.R. & Cole, W.A. (1976) The sickness impact profile: potential use of a health status instrument for physician training. *Journal of Medical Education*, 51, 283–287.

Mendoza, P. (2009) Experience of a Balint Group with medical students in Peru. *Journal of the Balint Society*, 37, 54.

Mezirow, J. (1991) *Transformative Dimensions of Adult Learning*. San Francisco: Jossey-Bass.

Moran, N. (2009) The Balint group and the doctor. *Journal of the Balint Society*, 37, 58–60.

Neumann, M., Edelhauser, F., Tauschel, D., Fischer, M.R., Wirtz, M., Woopen, C., Haramati, A., & Scheffer, C. (2011) Empathy decline and its reasons: a systematic review of studies with medical students and residents. *Academic Medicine*, 86, 996–1009.

Ney, P.G., Tam, W.W. & Maurice, W.L. (1990) Factors that determine medical student interest in psychiatry. *Australian and New Zealand Journal of Psychiatry*, 24, 65–76.

Nogueira-Martins, C.M.F., Nogueira-Martins, L.A. & Turato, E.R. (2006) Medical students' perceptions of their learning about the doctor–patient relationship: a qualitative study. *Medical Education*, 40, 322–328.

Nuffield Provincial Hospitals Trust (1985) *Talking with Patients. A Teaching Approach*. London.

Oatley K., Keltner D. & Jemkins J.M. (2006) *Understanding Emotions* (2nd edn). Malden, MA: Wiley-Blackwell.

Oldham, J.M., Sacks, M.H., Nininger, J.E., Blank, K. & Kaplan, R.D. (1983) Medical students: learning as primary therapists or as participants/observers in a psychiatric clerkship. *American Journal of Psychiatry*, 140, 1615–1618.

Orth, J.E., Stiles, W.B., Scherwitz, L., Henritus, D. & Vallbona, C. (1987) Patient exposition and provider explanation in routine interviews and hypertensive patients blood pressure control. *Health Psychology*, 6, 29–42.

Paar, G., Garbe, B. & Porstner, B. (1983) Content-analytical investigation of a junior Balint group. *Jahrbuch der Psychoanalyse*, 15, 290–316.

Parker, S. & Leggett, A. (2012) Teaching the clinical encounter in psychiatry: a trial of Balint groups for medical students. *Bulletin of the Royal Australian and New Zealand College of Psychiatrists*, 20, 343–347.

Pitkala, K.H. & Mantyranta, T. (2003) Professional socialization revised: medical students' own conceptions related to adoption of the future physician's role: a qualitative study. *Medical Teacher*, 25, 155–160.

Pitkala, K.H. & Mantyranta, T. (2004) Feelings related to first patient experiences in medical school: a qualitative study on students' personal experiences portfolios. *Patient Education and Counseling*, 54, 171–177.

Pollak, K.I., Arnold, R.M., Jeffreys, A.S., et al. (2007) Oncologist communication about emotion during visits with patients with advanced cancer. *Journal of Clinical Oncology*, 25, 5748–5752.

Powell, A. (1989) The nature of the group matrix. *Group Analysis*, 22, 271–281.

Prince, S. (1985) The role of a supervision group in learning to understand and treat patients in psychotherapy. In H.H. Wolff, W. Knauss & W. Brautigam (Eds), *First Steps in Psychotherapy*. Berlin: Springer-Verlag, pp. 96–99.

Reik, T. (1948) *Listening with the Third Ear: The Inner Experience of a Psychoanalyst*. New York: Grove Press.

Rhodes-Kropf, J., Carmody, S.S., Seltzer, D., Redinbaugh, E., Gadmer, N., Block, S.D. & Arnold, R.M. (2005) 'This is just too awful; I just can't believe I experienced that ...': Medical students' reactions to their 'most memorable' patient death. *Academic Medicine*, 80, 634–640.

Rizq, R. (2012) The ghost in the machine: IAPT and organizational melancholia. *British Journal of Psychotherapy*, 28, 319–335.

Roh, M.S., Hahm, B.J., Lee, D.H. & Suh, D.H. (2010) Psychometric properties of the Jefferson Scale of Physician Empathy among Korean medical students. *Teaching and Learning in Medicine*, 22, 167–171.

Roter, R. & Hall, J. (2006) *Doctors Talking with Patients/Patients Talking with Doctors: Improving Communication in Medical Visits*. London: Praeger.

Rucker, L. & Shapiro, J. (2003) Becoming a physician: students' creative projects in a third-year IM clerkship. *Academic Medicine*, 78, 391–397.

Salsberg, E., Rockey, P.H., Rivers, K.L., Brotherton, S.E. & Jackson, G.R. (2008) US residency training before and after the 1997 Balanced Budget act. *Journal of the American Medical Association*, 300, 1174–1180.

Schnabel, G.K., Hassard, T.H. & Kopelow, M.L. (1991) The assessment of interpersonal skills using standardised patients. *Academic Medicine*, 66, 34–36.

Schneider, D.E. & Tucker, R.K. (1992) Measuring communicative satisfaction in doctor–patient relations: The Doctor–Patient Communication Inventory. *Health Communication*, 4, 19–28.

Schonfield, J. & Donner, L. (1972) Student psychotherapists' specialty choices and changes in their perceptions of self and patient. *Journal of Medical Education*, 47, 645–651.

Schuffel, W. (1983) Can medical students acquire patient centred attitudes at medical schools? *Psychotherapy and Psychosomatics*, 40, 20–22.

Schulberg, H.C. & Burns, B.J. (1988) Mental disorders in primary care. *General Hospital Psychiatry*, 10, 79–87.

Scott, C.L., Martinovitch, Z., Lutz, W. & Lyons, J.S. (2005) The effect of therapist experience on psychotherapy outcomes. *Clinical Psychology and Psychotherapy*, 12, 417–426.

Shanafelt, T. & Dyrbye, L. (2012) Oncologist burnout: causes, consequences and responses. *Journal of Clinical Oncology*, 30, 1235–1241.

Shapiro, J. (2008) Walking a mile in their patients' shoes: empathy and othering in medical students' education. *Philosophy, Ethics and Humanities in Medicine*, 3, 10.

Shapiro, J. (2011) Does medical education promote professional alexithymia? A call for attending to the emotions of patients and self in medical training. *Academic Medicine*, 86, 326–332.

Shapiro, R.S., Simpson, D.E., Lawrence, S.L., Talsky, A.M., Subocinski, R.A. & Schiedermayer, D.L. (1989) A survey of sued and non sued physicians and suing patients. *Archives of Internal Medicine*, 149, 2190–2196.

Shapiro, S.M., Lancee, W.J. & Richards-Bentley, C. (2009) Evaluation of a communication skills program for first-year medical students at the University of Toronto. *BMC Medical Education*, 9, 11.

Sheehan, K.H., Sheehan, D.V., White, K., Leibovitz, A. & Balwin, D.C. Jr. (1990) A pilot study of medical student 'abuse': student perceptions of mistreatment and misconduct in the medical school. *Journal of the American Medical Association*, 263, 533–537.

Shoenberg, P.J. (1992) The Student Psychotherapy Scheme at the University College and Middlesex School of Medicine: Its role in helping medical students to learn about the doctor/patient relationship. *Journal of the Balint Society*, 20, 10–14.

Shoenberg, P. (2007) *Psychosomatics. The Uses of Psychotherapy*. Basingstoke: Palgrave.

Shoenberg, P. (2012) Students and their patients. Evaluating the UCL student Balint groups. *Journal of the Balint Society*, 40, 21–26.

Shoenberg, P. & Suckling, H. (2004) A Balint group for medical students at Royal Free and University College School of Medicine. *Journal of the Balint Society*, 32, 20–23.

Silver, H.K. & Glicken, A.D. (1990) Medical student abuse: incidence, severity, and significance. *Journal of the American Medical Association*, 263, 527–532.

Silverman, J., Kurtz, S. & Draper, J. (2005) *Skills for Communicating with Patients* (2nd edn). Oxford: Radcliffe Publishing.

Silverman, J. (2009) Teaching communication skills: a mainstream activity or just a minority sport? *Patient Education and Counseling*, 76, 361–67.

Simpson, M., Buckman, R., Stewart, M., Maguire, P., Lipkin, M., Novack, D. & Till, J. (1991) Doctor-patient communication: the Toronto Consensus Statement. *British Medical Journal*, 303, 1385–1387.

Simpson, M.A. (1980) *Psycholinguistics in Clinical Practice: the Languages of Illness and Healing*. New York: Irvington.

Sinclair, S. (1997) *Making Doctors: An Institutional Apprenticeship (Explorations in Anthropology)*. Oxford: Berg.

Smith, A., Juraskova, I., Butow, P., Miguel, C., Lopez, A.L., Chang, S., Brown, R. & Bernhard, J. (2011) Sharing vs. caring – the relative impact of sharing decisions versus managing emotions on patient outcomes. *Patient Education and Counseling*, 82, 233–239.

Smith, S., Hanson, J.L., Tewksbury, L.R., Christy, C., Talib, N.J., Harris, M.A., Beck, G.L. & Wolf, F.M. (2007) Teaching patient communication skills to medical students: a review of randomized controlled trials. *Evaluation and the Health Professions*, 30, 3–21.

Sollner, W., Maurer, G., Mark-Stemberger, B. & Wesiack, W. (1992) Characteristics and problems of Balint groups with medical students. *Psychotherapie, Psychosomatik, Medizinische Psychologie*, 42, 302–307.

Sturgeon, D. (1983) Development and organisation of the student-psychotherapy teaching scheme at University College Hospital. In H.H. Wolff, W. Knauss & W. Brautigam (Eds), *First Steps in Psychotherapy*. Berlin: Springer-Verlag, pp. 28–33.

Sturgeon, D. (1986) Outcome variables for medical students who take on psychotherapy patients. In J. H. Lacey and D.A. Sturgeon (Eds), *Proceedings of the 15th European Conference on Psychosomatic Research*. London: John Libbey, pp. 363–366.

Suckling, H. (2005) What do medical students discuss in Balint groups? International Balint Conference of the Romanian Balint Society.

Sung, A.D., Collins, M.E., Smith, A.K., Sanders, A.M., Quinn, M.A., Block, S.D. & Arnold, R.M. (2009) Crying: experiences and attitudes of third year medical students and interns. *Teaching and Learning in Medicine*, 21, 180–187.

Tamblyn, R., Abrahamowicz, M., Dauphinee, D., Wenghofer, E., Jacques, A., Klass, D., Smee, S., Blackmore, D., Winslade, N., Girard, N., Du Berger, R., Bartman, I., Buckeridge, D.L. & Hanley, J.A. (2007) Physician scores on a national clinical skills examination as predictors of complaints to medical regulatory authorities. *Journal of the American Medical Association*, 298, 993–1001.

Taveira, D.L.R., Freitas, F.G.M., Cerveira de Souza, L., Adorno, P.N., Carvalho, I., Lago, L. & Branco, R.F.G.R. (2010) Balint groups in the medical school of the Pontifical Catholic University of Goias: report of an educational experience. *Journal of the Balint Society*, 38, 9–12.

Thomas, K., Ellis, A., Konrad, T., Holzer, C. & Morrisset, J. (2009) County level estimates of mental health professional shortage in the United States. *Psychiatry Services*, 60, 1323–1328.

Thomson, L. & Dave, S. (2011) The organization of undergraduate teaching. In T. Brown & J. Eagles (Eds), *Teaching Psychiatry to Undergraduates*. London: Royal College of Psychiatrists, pp. 38–51.

Titchener, E.B. (1909) *Lectures on the Experimental Psychology of the Thought-Processes*. New York: Macmillan.

Torppa, M.A., Makkonen, E., Martenson, C. & Pitkala, K.H. (2008) A qualitative analysis of student Balint groups in medical education: contexts and triggers of case presentations and discussion themes. *Patient Education Counseling*, 72, 5–11.

Tredgold, R.F. (1962) The integration of psychiatric teaching into the curriculum. *Lancet*, 1, 1344–1347.

Tsimtsiou, Z., Kerasidou, O., Efstathiou, N., Papaharitou, S., Hatzimouratidis, K. & Hatzichristou, D. (2007) Medical students' attitudes to patient-centred care: a longitudinal survey. *Medical Education*, 41, 146–153.

Turner, A.L. (2005) Making space for the doctor–patient relationship through Balint training in the first year of medical school. In L. Karlsberg, T.N. Ronnas & H. Sjostrom (Eds), *Balint Work in a Time of Change and Crisis in the Health Care System. Proceedings of the 14th International Balint Congress*, Stockholm. Stockholm: Reproprint, pp. 42–45.

van Middendorp, H., Lumley, M.A., Jacobs, J.W., Bijlisma, J.W. & Grenen, R. (2010) The effects of anger and sadness on clinical pain reports and experimentally induced pain thresholds in women with and without fibromyalgia. *Arthritis Care Research*, 62, 1370–1376.

von Fragstein, M., Silverman, J., Cushing, A., Quilligan, S., Salisbury, H. & Wiskin, C. on behalf of the UK Council for Clinical Communication Skills Teaching in Undergraduate Medical Education (2008) UK consensus statement on the content of communication curricula in undergraduate medical education. *Medical Education*, 42, 1100–1107.

West, A. (2002) Letter to the editor. *British Medical Journal*, 324.

Whitehouse, C.R. (2009) The teaching of communication skills in United Kingdom medical schools. *Medical Education*, 25, 311–318.

Wolf, T.M., Balson, P.M., Faucett, J.M. & Randall, H.M. (1989) A retrospective study of attitude change during medical education. *Medical Education*, 23, 19–23.

Wolff, H., Bateman, A. & Sturgeon, D. (1990) Dedication in *UCH Textbook of Psychiatry*. London: Duckworth, p. x.

Yakeley, J.W., Shoenberg, P. & Heady, A. (2004) Who wants to do psychiatry: the influence of a student psychotherapy scheme – a ten year retrospective study. *Psychiatric Bulletin*, 28, 208–212.

Yakeley, J., Shoenberg, P., Morris, R., Majid, S. & Sturgeon, D. (2011) A randomized controlled trial to evaluate 2 psychodynamic teaching approaches for medical students to learn about the doctor patient relationship. *The Psychiatrist*, 35, 308–313.

Zalidis, S. (2001) *A General Practitioner, his Patients and their Feelings. Exploring the Emotions behind Physical Symptoms*. London: Free Association Books.

Zenasni, F., Boujut, E., Woerner, A. & Sultan, S. (2012) Burnout and empathy in primary care: three hypotheses. *British Journal of General Practice*, 62, 346–347.

Zimny, G.H. & Sata, L.S. (1986) Influence of factors before and during medical school on choice of psychiatry as a specialty. *American Journal of Psychiatry*, 143, 77–80.

Index